LIVING WITH HERPES

Deborah P. Langston, M.D.

LIVING
WITH HERPES

The Comprehensive and Authoritative Guide to the Causes, Symptoms, and Treatment of Herpes Virus Illnesses

A DOLPHIN BOOK

Doubleday & Company, Inc., Garden City, New York 1983

Library of Congress Cataloging in Publication Data

Langston, Deborah P.
Living with herpes.

"A Dolphin book."
Bibliography: p. 175
Includes index.
1. Herpesvirus diseases.   I. Title.
RC147.H6P38   1983   616.9′25
ISBN 0-385-18410-7
Library of Congress Catalog Card Number 82–45627

To my children, Talcott and Wyndy, and to those who work to free us of herpes in making the world safe for all children.

PREFACE

Until recently most people had never heard of herpes virus. Even doctors were familiar only with cold sores and shingles. In the past few years, however, it has become clear that herpes infections are much more widespread than had been thought. There is, in fact, a worldwide herpes epidemic.

This book has been written for the public, who have heard about, read about, worried about and, in many cases, had to deal directly with herpetic illness. It tells which herpes virus does what, and whether or not it is venereal in nature. Contrary to much current opinion *"having herpes" is not synonymous with having venereal disease*—far from it. But that, of course, is what concerns us all. Some, but not all, herpes viruses are the cause of this international epidemic which is still not under control and will not be under control until we all understand the "rules and regulations" of living safely and successfully with this virus in us or near us.

Many people have helped me in writing this book. Not least are the thousands who have written to me these past few years asking about our new antiherpetic drugs and where they could find information on and medical help for herpes, or, seeking emotional support, just wanting to tell me how unhappy or frightened they were. They were the main stimulus for the undertaking of this manuscript.

Elaine Spaulding, Ph.D., A.C.S.W., provided constant kind support and advice in the discussion of the psychological impact herpes has had on virtually everyone. Loretta Barrett of Doubleday has been a wonderfully encouraging and helpful editor, and I thank Anne Jardim for her contribution in this regard.

I acknowledge also the tireless assistance given me by Mary Lou Moar, Karen Cirisi, Patricia Geary and Pauline Calliste at the Eye Research Institute of Retina Foundation in Boston. Without the help of all these people and countless others too numerous to name, this book might still be in preparation.

CONTENTS

LIVING WITH HERPES

Table I: Estimated Frequency and Location of Oral (Herpes Type-1) and Genital (Herpes Type-2) Infections

Location of Primary or Recurrent Disease	Most Frequent Herpes Type	Estimated No. Cases/Year in U.S.A.
Primary		
Mouth	95% type-1	500,000
Eye	95% type-1	Unknown
Recurrent		
Mouth	95% type-1	98 million
Eye	95% type-1	280,000–300,000
Primary		
Genital	60–90% type-2	20,000–500,000
Fingers	80% (?) type-2	Unknown
Recurrent		
Genital	70–85% type-2 15–30% type-1	3–9 million
Fingers	often type-2	Unknown

1. AN OVERVIEW OF THE HERPES PROBLEM: HOW TO LIVE WITH IT, HOW TO AVOID IT

"Herpes virus* type-1 occurs above the waist and herpes virus type-2 occurs below the waist." That statement was true a few years ago when herpes simplex type-1 just infected the mouth and

* Herpes virus may also be written as "herpesvirus."

eyes and herpes simplex type-2 infected the genitals. But with our new sexual freedom, our ways of living and making love to one another have changed greatly. And with that change, where and how frequently we find the two types of herpes virus in our bodies has changed. But type-1 and type-2 are far from the only herpes viruses that affect our lives. If you have any herpes virus in you—and, as Table I indicates, the chances are very high that you do—you are just one of millions of people carrying this organism. *This does not mean, however, that you will ever come down with an herpetic illness, nor does it mean you have venereal disease.* Nearly two out of three people who have some form of herpes virus in them never have any problem with it. But one third do and could pass it on. Just learning a few facts about herpes can either help prevent you from catching it or, if you have it now, help you avoid spreading it as you learn to live successfully with herpes.

Only the specific virus and where you get your attacks in your body separates you into one diagnostic group or another. Some groups have more worrisome illnesses than others, but all may be treated and the effects of disease, whether physical or psychological, made much less.

This book has been written to tell you about the many diseases that the herpes simplex virus, the herpes zoster virus, and the cytomegalovirus produce, what they look like, what they can and can not do to you and to those you love, what you and your doctor can do to help you in understanding it, to live successfully with it, and to treat it. Toward this end, I have included many true personal experiences and medical case reports. This will not only let you know that you are not alone in your reactions to your illness but tell you how others have coped successfully with it. As you will see, some of these experiences have had good and some have had sad endings, but there is a lesson you can learn from each. Remember, also, that some of these experiences took place before we had emotional support groups for people with herpes, before the medical community had a true awareness of the extent of herpetic illness, and before the existence of any of the new specific treatments which are just now being developed and marketed.

Today we hear about herpes all the time—on television, on the radio, in the newspapers and magazines. We hear that there is an epidemic under way, that once the virus infects us it remains in us as a threat to us and our loved ones for the rest of our lives. But what is this epidemic? Is it just one kind of illness or does it take many forms? Is there more than one kind of herpes and are we confusing illnesses caused by one herpes virus type with that caused by another? The overall answer, as I mentioned above, is that there are indeed many forms of illness caused by different members of the herpes virus family and, yes, we are confusing the illnesses each can produce. Most people do not realize that cold sores, genital ulcers, mononucleosis, chicken pox, and shingles are all caused by herpes viruses. Each and every one of these may be said to occur in epidemic proportions in this country if we go by sheer numbers alone. But that is not how we really define an epidemic in our population. It is not the number of cases themselves but an unexpected or radical rise in the number that constitutes an epidemic. There has, in fact, been no radical change in the percentage of our population that has chicken pox, cold sores, herpes of the eyes, viral brain infection, or herpetic "heartburn and indigestion." The change has occurred in only one segment of the herpes virus family: those infections which are related to our lovemaking and sexual activity; only the incidence of venereal herpes has risen.

Herpes infections "below the waist" were so unusual just fifteen years ago that few doctors, much less their patients, knew what it was when they contracted it. Until the present epidemic, what relatively little genital herpes there was was caused by herpes simplex type-2 and so *type-2 became synonymous with venereal herpes. Type-1 infections seemed fairly confined to the facial region and were named oral herpes.* But in the 1960s our world seemed to go wild and society exploded into a bevy of activities which went against all the so-called "established rules." This resulted in not only an absolute increase in sexual behavior but in the expansion and exploration of many different forms of love-making—which included conventional genital-to-genital sex, plus a variety of oral-anal-genital contacts. Certainly, part of this increase in sexual function was due to the development of the contraceptive pill, but part seems due to the general stresses of the times. Whether it was the Vietnam war, the unstable economy, disillusionment with our government, or drugs, no one can say;

most likely it was a function of all four, and then some. The net result was the same, however: increased stress, increased sexual contact without the protection of mechanical barrier contraceptives and viricidal gels, and the great variety in forms of contact gave the herpes simplex viruses their chance. Type-2 got to the face and type-1 got to the genital area, both in far greater frequency than either had done previously. But regardless of which type of genital herpes someone had, a pattern of recurrent infection often occurred. The virus simply slept in the body between attacks; it never really died. Fortunately, only about one third of all people who have genital infections suffer recurring disease and, of this group, a significant number actually have a decreasing frequency of attacks with the passage of time. Nonetheless, what was initially a relatively small number of genital infections became enough to spread the disease far and wide, once coupled with changes in sexual activity in the population.

We now know that approximately twenty million people have type-2 genital herpes; nearly one out of every ten people, a figure which does not even include those who have oral herpes (type-1) infecting the genital region. If only one third of type-2 herpes-infected people were to pass their virus on to one other person in the next year, nearly twenty-seven million people would have the illness. This would be close to 15 percent of the country and would represent an increase of roughly 40 percent over already existing type-2 infections.

The potential rate at which genital infection can be spread by people not sure of how to manage their illness properly is one of the major reasons why herpes is so frightening. Not knowing how to protect yourself from getting it is another—but these are only two of many reasons.

What other differences to our lives has the spread of this genital infection made? The psychological impact has been tremendous and the enormity of the problem greatly enhanced by the fact that widespread ignorance of what herpes is all about has managed to stay well ahead of the spread of useful medical information and reassurance. The medical profession itself was caught short, both in realizing how great the problem had become and in developing treatment for it. It was not uncommon for a patient with recurring genital blisters to seek many medical opinions, at great expense of time and money, before a diagnosis was finally made. Even then, he or she was often told nothing could be done for it. That patient would, very likely, discourage any friends with the same illness from seeking medical advice. It appeared such an exercise in futility. This, of course, would only further delay doctors' realizing how rapidly the genital infection was spreading and thus delay the all-out effort now under way to tell people how very much can already be done for herpes infections and to develop new treatment for it.

By the late 1970s, millions upon millions of people discovered they had genital herpes infections and were plunged into a wide variety of emotional reactions to the unexpected changes in their lives. Initially, most were outraged and angry at the person who gave them the infection. Those who did not know where they got it were simply bewildered. But as the anger and bewilderment passed, new and equally troublesome emotions set in. For fear of spreading the infection themselves, many people withdrew from society, and with social isolation came depression and guilt. Some felt they were being punished for doing something which is a perfectly normal human need. But in their isolation they were not cut off from hearing many false rumors about genital herpes. They heard that they would spread the disease any time they had sex, that it was dangerous ever to become pregnant or to have a baby, that they might go blind, suffer brain damage, or develop cancer, and that there was no treatment. They seemed forever condemned to live alone, wondering when the next attack would come.

And then things began to change. The number of people with herpes infections passed a critical breaking point. The medical profession, government health agencies, and the pharmaceutical industry realized what was happening and set out to make things better. Study after study was done to find out just how widespread the illness was, how people were coping or not coping with it, what the natural untreated courses of the infections were, when it was all right to have sexual activity and when it was not, how to make it perfectly safe for a woman to have a baby, and whether herpes, by itself, really causes cancer.

In addition to the concerted efforts by the medical profession and pharmaceutical industry to bring genital herpes under control, the people themselves began to organize in forming self-help groups. These groups range in size from just a few to hundreds of members and now exist in or near almost every major city. They are task-oriented, focusing exclusively on the members' common problem: genital herpes. Through regular meetings with other people with herpes, with or without the presence of a professional social worker, psychiatrist, or psychologist, members of these groups exchange useful and supportive information. Those who know more than others pass their information on, but most importantly, everyone discovers that he or she is not alone in coping with the virus. The stress and loneliness of self-imposed social isolation comes to an end. Guilt and anger are relieved. New friendships are formed by many at these meetings and other members bring close friends or lovers who do not have herpes themselves but who want to understand more about it for the sake of their own relationships. Members of the medical profession serve as advisers and pass on new information as it becomes available. As knowledge of how normally and successfully one can live despite herpes grows, confidence builds. Ultimately, many members of these organizations no longer feel the need for continued support through task-oriented groups. They have learned the facts about herpes and how to manage their infection well or how to protect themselves from it. No one could ever say that their lives had not changed in unexpected ways, but they had, through knowledge and emotional support, come to terms with their illness and could go back to the business of a normal life. Only a few new rules had been added.

There are, of course, yet other effects that genital herpes has had on many lives. Pregnancy and birth most certainly are high on the list. Women of childbearing age will be those who worry most about the effects of such infection, but any caring man should also bear his share of responsibility in following guidelines that will assure an uncomplicated pregnancy, a safe delivery, and a healthy baby. We now have quite an accurate knowledge of the behavior of genital herpes through the course of pregnancy and excellent diagnostic tools which support the guidelines of successful management both preterm and after the baby has arrived.

Fortunately, herpes infection in a new baby is now a rare event because of our extensive experience with care of expectant mothers who have genital herpes infections. But, on occasion, the virus does gain access to the newborn. It is estimated that this occurs in one to five out of every ten thousand births. The personal case reports presented in this book span the period before and after we knew what to look for, and what to do about it in successfully treating these children. You will learn, in reviewing these chapters, what precautions should be taken before and after delivery to protect your baby not only from genital virus but from oral herpes as well. The signs of early herpes infection, whether type-2 from the birth canal or type-1 from your mouth, are the same and should be known to you so that effective treatment may be started immediately upon recognition. But most importantly, you will learn not to be afraid to love and handle your baby.

While pregnancy is probably the main concern of most women with genital herpes, we are all aware of the reports that cancer in the birth canal may be caused by this virus. There is some scientific foundation for this statement, but the critical facts are that there are many more women with genital cancer who have never had herpes than those who do have the infection, that herpes is probably only one of many factors needed to cause malignant changes in the cells, and that, with knowledge of how often you should visit your gynecologist and what simple tests should be done, any early cancer will be diagnosed and is 100 percent curable.

While herpes simplex types 1 or 2 are of greatest concern because they are the cause of a widespread epidemic of genital infections, *there are many other nonvenereal forms of herpetic disease* which serve as the source of worrisome rumors which need clarification. These are discussed in greater detail in this book. In brief, we can say that type-1 is most often responsible for infections of the skin, especially around the face, the mouth and digestive tract, the eyes, the brain, and even the joints (arthritis). These vary in frequency from very common, as in cold sores of the mouth, to very rare, as in arthritis. Each of these has its own importance in terms of recognition, management, knowing what treatment is already available, and what to expect in the future. Type-2 is most often responsible for herpetic neuralgia, especially of the legs, infection of the fingers, and meningitis (infection of the membranes surrounding the brain). All of these occur relatively infrequently, but it is important for you to know the signs of each and their significance in terms of how they are best managed.

If herpes simplex is of concern as a major public health problem which we should all know about, why then is it important for us to learn about herpes zoster virus? It is because zoster, otherwise known as shingles and caused by the all-familiar chicken pox virus, mimics in many ways the illnesses and complications of the herpes simplex virus. Patients with shingles are sometimes told simply that they have "herpes" and then live unnecessarily in a state of confusion over their illness. Zoster can cause a blistering rash indistinguishable from simplex, a rash which may involve any site on the body, including the genitalia—but it is not a venereal illness and it does not recur in a basically healthy person. It can, however, cause a severe neuralgia which may often be prevented by early appropriate treatment. Zoster may also affect the eye in a chronic illness which must be treated much the way herpes simplex of the eye is managed. Familiarity with the differences and similarities between the two herpes virus infections can help you in knowing both what should be done and what you might expect in the future course of the illness.

We come, then, to the last major form of herpetic infection and find ourselves faced with yet another epidemic. Cytomegalovirus (or CMV) is a herpes virus normally found in about one of every two to four people. Until recently, it has not constituted a major public health problem. About two years ago, however, something changed and an epidemic of CMV infection appeared in the gay population, almost exclusively among young men. Since that time, some cases have been reported in the heterosexual population. This illness is one that needs early diagnosis and therapy, as its untreated course is one of progressive recurrences not only of CMV infection but superimposed bacterial infection and a high rate of a cancer which is usually very rare. The reasons why this epidemic has appeared now and why it started in the gay population are gradually being worked out, but the answers are not yet complete. Nonetheless, the probable contributing factors should be known to all of us, as none of them are confined to any one group of people.

We have reviewed briefly the background and problems of the

herpes simplex epidemic and the illnesses caused by other members of this virus family which, in one way or other, affect each of us. What about where we stand today in terms of developing definitive treatment for the herpes viruses? This is discussed in greater detail later under appropriate sections in this book, but an overview of the development of antiviral treatment may put the current relative scarcity of drugs into perspective and give us all hope for the future.

Antiviral therapy is only now coming of age and is focused particularly on the herpes virus family.

Just how far we have come in developing treatment for infection by a member of this virus family can be seen if we compare our situation now with the development of antibiotics for bacterial infections. Just forty years ago, we had only the sulfas available. During World War II, penicillin was made available to our troops and then released for everyone's use around 1945. That one drug alone revolutionized our concept of how to treat bacterial disease. Penicillin prevented the growth of the bacterial cell wall and thus defeated the infection by preventing new bacteria from maturing. We understood the mechanism by which penicillin worked, and as we learned more mechanisms of bacterial growth we developed more and better drugs for treating them. The tetracyclines interfere with certain bacterial enzymes, yet another mechanism for killing bacteria. Since the tetracyclines, virtually hundreds of new broad-spectrum antibiotics have been developed for treatment of all kinds of infections. Many of these drugs were developed in the late 1940s and early 1950s. The pharmaceutical industry can and does now synthesize the majority of the most potent antibiotics; very few come from natural sources, such as the molds from which penicillin and tetracycline were first isolated.

Such synthesis of drugs played a prominent role in the development of the first antiviral drugs. Anticancer agents were being made and tested in the early 1960s, when it was discovered that they not only interfered with enzymes necessary to keep cancer cells alive but with enzymes that herpes viruses needed too. At that time, genital infection was a minor if not totally ignored problem, but herpes was recognized as (and still is) the most common infectious cause of impaired vision in this country. The first antiviral drug, IDU, was developed as an eye drop to treat herpes simplex ulcers of the front of the eye and it worked beautifully. Unfortunately, IDU was too toxic to be given by injection or orally and did not penetrate well enough to be used on the skin. Within a very few years of IDU's commercial marketing, another drug, vidarabine (Ara-A), was developed. This drug is relatively nontoxic and, therefore, can be used as an ointment for herpes of the eye and intravenously to treat herpes infections of the brain. The latter illness was previously an almost uniformly fatal disease. As you will see later in this book, Ara-A is also of use in other herpes infections, including those of the newborn baby and in shingles. Unfortunately, Ara-A did not penetrate well either and was not effective on the skin or genitalia.

It was about the time that Ara-A was being developed that it was discovered that there were two forms of herpes simplex virus: type-1, which was found around the face, and type-2, which was found in the genital area. In looking back, we can see how very elementary our knowledge of herpes was just fifteen years ago. We hardly knew there was more than one type of herpes simplex, much less the intimate mechanics of the viral life cycle, information crucial to the development of more specific and less toxic drugs. In fact, the next antiherpes drug to be marketed was another eye drop, trifluridine, a superb ocular drug but again, too toxic to be given orally or by injection.

By the mid- and late 1970s, however, we not only knew a great deal about the virus life cycle but could begin to synthesize drugs which acted only against herpes enzymes and were, therefore, not poisonous to the person taking them. In addition, the existence of the genital herpes epidemic was being recognized in the medical community and by the pharmaceutical industry. Tremendous pressure for effective treatment was brought to bear by a public made ever more aware of the problem by the lay press and television media. The media had themselves only recently recognized what was happening and how important it was as a public health dilemma. Several agencies of the National Institutes of Health declared herpes one of the, if not *the,* most important infectious problem of the decade and funded its research accordingly. The pharmaceutical industry poured millions of dollars into developing better drugs and continues to do so. The rewards from all this effort are now beginning to come in. The first drug for treatment of some forms of genital and skin herpes has already been marketed; it is acyclovir. Not far behind is another drug, bromo-vinyldeoxyuridine, abbreviated BVDU. This drug is not as effective against type-2 herpes as type-1, but this in no way diminishes its potential use in genital herpes infections. One out of every three genital herpes patients under the age of twenty-four—and there are millions of them—has type-1, not type-2, "below the waist." These people may be expected to respond well to therapy with BVDU. In addition, both BVDU and acyclovir may be given as pills and both are effective against many other members of the herpes virus family.

So where do we stand in our comparison with the development of antivirals versus antibiotics? It would seem that we are somewhere in the late 1940s. The first good drugs have appeared, but better ones are on the way. If it is anything like the story of antibiotics, we shall have highly effective therapy or preventive vaccines within an encouragingly short period of time.

While there is great hope for the future, then, we do live in the present and must cope with the problems herpes presents using the tools available today. In order to know which tools to use, we must understand what the separate forms of herpetic illness are and which virus causes them. This book has been written toward this end in an effort to help you understand and live successfully with the herpes viruses.

2. FOUR PEOPLE WITH HERPES

Herpes viruses may cause many different kinds of disease. The following stories are typical of people who were in trouble because they became infected with a member of this family of germs. One or more of these cases may sound familiar.

Case 1: Susan W. is a twenty-year-old college student who had been steadily dating a classmate, Jason R., for three months. Shortly after their second date, Jason began to urge Susan to sleep with him. In all fairness to her, however, he

told her that he had once had an attack of herpes blistering
in his genital area but had had no evidence of any further infection in two years. They began to have intercourse several
times a week without using a condom. Susan was on the Pill.
One month later, she suddenly developed a fever, generalized
muscle aching, and clear watery blisters appeared over her
entire genital region. Because of the severe pain and frightening appearance of the blisters, she went to the university
health center where, after an internal and external examination of her genital and vaginal area, the physician told her
that she had herpes virus, probably a first infection. It would
get better but could return at any time. She left the health
center in a state of confusion. She had had sexual relations
only with Jason. How could she have caught the infection
from him when he had had no sign of the disease in more
than two years? Could she give it to other people now?
Would it affect her babies in the future? What should she do
now?

Case 2: Dorothy L. had had a very active sex life with
many partners since the age of eighteen. As far as she knew,
however, she had never contracted disease from any of them.
Dorothy married at twenty-one and became pregnant within
a few months. One week before she entered the hospital to
have her baby, a small cluster of blisters appeared on the
index finger of her right hand. They ruptured into unsightly
red ulcers, so she covered them with a bandage. She did not
tell her obstetrician because it did not seem important.
Dorothy was delivered through her birth canal of an apparently healthy six-pound boy. The day after delivery, she
ran a slight fever and was put on antibiotics. The baby
seemed fine. Then, when he was five days old, her son suddenly stopped feeding and became very sleepy. Within a matter of hours, he had the first of many convulsions. Examination revealed an ulcer in his left eye and watery blisters on
both cheeks. The astute pediatrician diagnosed congenital
herpes virus of the eye and brain. He started the baby on antiviral and anticonvulsant treatment immediately. Within a
few days, the baby became more alert and the blisters and

eye ulcer healed. The infant was sent home three weeks later, but the pediatrician told Dorothy that it would be some time before they would know if the child would develop normally. Dorothy wondered where the virus came from. The doctor said it was in her birth canal. She did not think she had ever had herpes—or had she?

Case 3: Mary C. had dropped out of high school at the age of fourteen. Two years later, she was working in the kitchen of a large hotel where she met many men and had many sexual encounters. By the time she was twenty, Mary had genital herpes and she knew it; she had had at least fifteen attacks in the previous three years. The attacks lasted only a few days and she could live with it; she just didn't see any of her boyfriends on those days. It would be bad if she passed the virus along to people for whom she felt great affection.

Twenty-two years later, Mary had a new problem. Her gynecologist had taken a Pap smear on routine physical exam a few days before. He had just called to tell her that she had cancer—cancer deep in her vagina on the cervix. This was where her herpes had smoldered for twenty-two years. Was there any connection? She would ask her doctor; he was admitting her to the hospital next week. The surgery, he said, would cure her.

Case 4: David G. was forty-eight years old when he went to visit his young nephew who had chicken pox. Ten days later, David awoke with severe pain over the right side of his head; it hurt to touch his scalp and there seemed to be a red rash over his forehead and right eyelid. Two days later, a crop of watery blisters erupted over his right forehead and eyelid. The vision in his right eye blurred and intense shooting pain made him feel as if that side of his head were splitting open. He had "shingles." David was treated by an eye doctor with antiviral ointments and cortisone (anti-inflammatory) medication. The blisters broke, crusted over, and finally healed, leaving him with pitted scars on his forehead, scarring of the right eye which made vision poor, and the pain which continued on and on. He lost weight because he couldn't eat and he lost his job because he couldn't work. David consulted many physicians who could do little for him. Finally, he found a neurologist who gave him a pill to take four times daily. The doctor told him that this pill usually was very effective in controlling the pain, but that if it did not work he would have to consider a surgical procedure to kill the nerve. David was in luck; the drug worked.

3. THE HERPES VIRUSES: THEIR NATURE AND PLACE IN SOCIETY

Viruses

Viruses are widespread common germs which may cause anything from a mild nose cold to severe liver infection. They differ from bacterial germs in that they are too small to be seen with an ordinary microscope; they can grow only inside living body cells and they are not sensitive to any of the antibiotics that we use to kill bacteria. These three factors often make it more difficult to diagnose viral disease and to treat it. The antiviral drugs that we do have available today may make a patient sicker than his disease if not used properly. Fortunately, medical research and the drug industry are changing all of this as new, effective, and less toxic medications are being developed.

The Herpes Virus Family

More than fifty different kinds of herpes viruses are scattered throughout the animal kingdom. They produce the familiar "cold sore" in monkeys and infect at least thirty other species of animals, including dogs, cats, rodents, poultry, large farm animals, fish, and reptiles. This results in a variety of throat, lung, and skin afflictions, and, in some cases, cancerous disease.

There are four major members of the herpes family that infect humans: 1) Herpes simplex types 1 and 2 cause the vast majority of diseases discussed in this book, including infections of the genitals, skin, eyes, brain, and newborn baby. Seven out of ten people over the age of five years and nine out of ten over fifty years have some form of herpes simplex in them. Fortunately, only about 30 to 40 percent of them actually have any herpetic illness. 2) Herpes zoster, also known as "shingles," is identical to chicken pox and causes an often painful local infection of the skin or eye. Because its name includes the word "herpes," it is often confused with herpes simplex, but the two viruses cause different diseases and are treated differently. Chicken pox-zoster virus infects nearly 100 percent of the population. Chicken pox is usually quite harmless, but shingles can be a problem. About one to two million people come down with this illness each year. Zoster will be discussed to help you in understanding the differences between the infections. 3) Cytomegalovirus (CMV), another human herpes virus, may rarely cause severe disease in babies before birth, resulting in children who are blind and mentally retarded. In adults, this infection is thought to be a reactivation of an old "harmless" infection originally picked up around the time of birth and is usually seen in patients who are chronically ill from disease (such as leukemia) or in kidney transplant patients. It is strongly associated with a devastating illness now sweeping the homosexual population. CMV will be discussed in a separate section. 4) Epstein-Barr virus, the fourth prominent member of the herpes family, is now known to cause mononucleosis or "the kissing disease." It also causes certain types of fatal cancer (lymphoma) in Africans. Because Epstein-Barr virus is not yet recognized as a major problem throughout this country, it will not be discussed in much greater detail in this book.

The History of Herpes—From Ancient Confusion to Modern Enlightenment

Before we enter further discussion of our present knowledge of herpetic illness, it would be useful for you to have some understanding of how long, how badly, and how well we have struggled with this problem in the past. As you will see, it took the medical world a considerable time to come to grips with this virus family; close to 90 percent of our diagnostic and treatment capabilities were developed within the last half century alone.

The infectious organisms which afflict all of us at one time or other are as old as life itself. Germs, such as viruses and bacteria, are so simple in structure and function that they appeared on earth as the first forms of life at least two and possibly three billion years ago—long before the first land animals. We might even think of these tiny organisms in their earliest days as germs in search of disease. And create disease they did, but not immediately or in epidemic form. Many human germs probably evolved along with the human race in a mutually nondestructive relationship for thousands of years. Epidemic disease, both venereal and nonvenereal, appears to have started as humans began to organize socially in larger and more complex, close-quartered groups. Rapid spread of illness is the result of an accident of nature, an upset in the balance of life through the introduction of a new germ into a population not accustomed to living at peace with it; there is no immunity against it. It is clear that today our incessant meddling with the earth's ecology has put us into a state of instability which affects us not only physically but emotionally, and both of these factors have their effect on the herpes viruses.

Assuming, then, that some forms of herpes viruses have, like most other families of germs, existed on the earth for millions of years, why are we only now becoming so aware of its presence? Didn't they cause disease among earlier civilizations as well? The answer is yes. But if we are confused about this virus family today with all modern technology available to us, imagine what it must have been like centuries ago when reports of herpetic disease first began to appear inscribed on tablets, scrawled on parchment, or ultimately cranked out on the early printing presses.

"Herpes" derives its name from the Greek word *herpein,* which means to creep or to crawl. There are, however, many diseases which seem to creep or crawl across the body. In their confusion, the ancient Greek physicians treating "herpes" over 2,000 years ago used this term with reference to virtually any lesion spreading across the skin. This included not only real herpes but cancer, tuberculosis of the skin, ringworm, bacterial infections, and eczema. Hippocrates, in his treatise *Epidemics,* probably gave the first recognizable descriptions of herpes simplex infection of the mouth in his patients who suffered "ardent fever, phrensy, and apthous infections of the mouth—" Intermittent fever and ulceration of the lips could also be involved. Similarly, he was probably the first to write on herpes zoster or shingles. In the *Corpus Hippocraticum,* he described herpetic sores in the groin which spread toward the flank and genital region (or could this have been a more severe form of genital herpes simplex?).

By the first century A.D., Rome had become a center of medical instruction. The great Roman scientist Celsus was familiar with some of the manifestations of what we now know as herpes. He described herpetic sores around the mouth in association with fever, cold sores, and the more serious ulcerating sores seen in children, for many, herpes simplex. Celsus also recognized shingles and gave it the name "zoster" from the Greek word meaning belt. Unfortunately, he failed to distinguish herpes from many other infections with a similar appearance.

Galen of Pergamon, a Greek physician of the second century A.D., whose writings were influential until the end of the Middle Ages, was in equal confusion where herpes was concerned. In his writings *Definitions* he described herpes in one chapter as a disease involving ulcers and in yet another chapter as a disease not always involving ulcers. He did at least argue that herpes was a very different disease from the bacterial infection erysipelas and stated that herpes was the less serious condition. In those ancient days, of course, that statement was true. There were no antibiotics available then for the cure of the bacterial infection; erysipelas was often fatal. Herpes at least "went away" spontaneously. Any person infected with herpes in modern times, however, might well question which is the more distressing condition.

In the centuries that followed, physicians gradually began to differentiate more accurately among all the diseases labeled herpes. Rembrandt, in his famous painting "The Anatomy Lesson," immortalized the seventeenth-century Dutch physician Nicholas Tulpius. Tulpius accurately described herpes zoster and recognized it as an infection definitely separable in identity.

Not long after Tulpius' descriptive essay on herpes zoster came the first of the English writings. James Cooke, an otherwise unheard-of country practitioner, wrote in his book *Mellificium Chirurgiae* a description of herpes simplex cold sores that would be recognizable to anyone today. "In herpes there's little pustules like to millet seeds. Heat, itching, after rubbing a little moistness, and little ulcers."*

Just forty years later, in the early eighteenth century, Dr. Daniel Turner clearly described and differentiated between the diseases herpes simplex and herpes zoster. Modern sufferers from either disease will recognize his observations as similar to their own. "The herpes is a choleric pustule breaking forth of the skin diversely, and accordingly receiving a diverse denomination. If they single, as they often do in the face, they arise with a sharp top and inflamed base: and having discharged a drop of matter they contain, the redness and pain go off and they dry away of themselves."* This is herpes simplex.

"There is another species of this disease, appearing in larger heaps of small pustules upon several parts of the body as the neck, breast, loyns, hips, and thighs; these are usually attended with a light fever and inflammation round about them, and rising up with white mattery heads, there succeeds a small round scab, resembling the millet seed from which the disease has borrowed the name of herpes milaris, being the same with that our people call shingles."* Unfortunately, while Turner's descriptions of the diseases are good, he fell into the same trap as did so many of his predecessors in using the diagnosis of herpes in nonherpetic disease. For Turner, the confusion lay in the inclusion of ringworm, a fungal infection, in the herpetic diseases. And like the teachings of his predecessors, his own misdiagnosis of ringworm as herpetic was widely taught and thus passed on to future generations of physicians until well into the mid-1800s.

In fact, physicians of the eighteenth and nineteenth centuries became totally bogged down in classifying and naming things, rather than advancing their knowledge of the cause and cure of disease. Thomas Bateman, in his *Delineations of Cutaneous Disease* (1817), classified no fewer than six different forms of herpes. One of these was zoster of the face, a second zoster of the chest, but there was no mention of zoster involving the abdomen, legs, or any other part of the body where it may appear. A third category was almost certainly ringworm and a fourth probably another type of fungus infection or an allergic inflammation of

* Juel-Jensen, B., and Maccallum, F. *Herpes Simplex Varicella and Zoster* (J. B. Lippincott Co., Philadelphia, 1972), pp. 1–5.

the blood vessels. But, in his fifth and sixth categories, this physician more than made up for the errors of his first four categories in his descriptions of "herpes labialis" (lips) and "herpes praeputialis" (genitals). Although the French physician Jean Astruc had first described involvement of the genitalia by herpes nearly one hundred years before Bateman's report, Bateman must be credited as being the first to recognize and to report the existence of two different forms of herpes simplex—oral and genital. Over the one hundred and sixty-five years since his publications, we have adhered to and proven the validity of his observations. But Bateman too had his great failing. He reported that no form of herpes was infectious!

During the remainder of the nineteenth century, physicians dug themselves still deeper into the quagmire of disease classification and subclassification, adding more and more confusion to their own understanding of the nature of herpetic disease. The only new contribution was a description by Ferdinand von Hebra, and later by his student Moritz Kaposi, of a particularly fulminant and widespread herpes infection of the skin. Eighty percent of the patients suffering this form of herpes simplex died. It is now known as Kaposi's varicelliform (chicken pox-like) eruption (not to be confused with Kaposi's sarcoma, a malignant tumor).

The twentieth century saw the birth of modern clinical medicine and with it came the age of enlightenment for herpetic disease. It is possible to mention by name only a few of the many investigators who have contributed to our present understanding of the illnesses caused by this virus family. By the 1920s, men like Gruter and Lowenstein had not only identified the herpes simplex virus as the infectious cause of cold sores around the mouth and scarring ulcers of the eye but had also successfully transferred the virus to the eyes of rabbits (who do not harbor herpes simplex in nature) and thus recreated the disease. By the 1930s, workers such as Lipschutz and Cowdry had established the first easy laboratory diagnostic tests to identify the clusters of herpes viruses in cell scrapings taken from patients' ulcers. As this technique involves only a simple staining procedure and an ordinary microscope, it is still used in many physicians' offices today. Other notable discoveries concerning herpes simplex made during the 1930s, '40s, and '50s included finding: 1) specific viral antibodies in the blood of almost all adults, indicating that almost all adults have been infected at some time in life; 2) herpes simplex infection as a cause of death in premature babies (probably genital virus picked up during passage through an infected birth canal); 3) herpes as a common cause of brain infection (encephalitis); and 4) herpes simplex as the most common viral infection of mankind in the United States, Europe, and Australia. The development of tissue culture by John Enders and his co-workers led to the ability to grow the viruses under laboratory control; new drugs could be tested in test tubes growing herpes.

Although it was suspected during much of this time that herpes of the face was caused by a virus biologically similar to but certainly not identical to herpes of the genital region, this momentous discovery was not actually made until the 1960s and early 1970s by scientists such as Shubladze, Chzhu-Shan, Schneweis, Nahmias, Amstey, and Roizman. During this same era, it was also found that although herpes zoster viruses looked identical to herpes simplex viruses under the great magnification of the electron microscopes, zoster was, by certain biochemical standards, really chicken pox virus.

Common Bonds Among Herpes Viruses

All herpes viruses look alike physically. They are medium-sized viruses with a central genetic core made of DNA surrounded by a protein cover. Around the cover is a fatty membrane which newly made viruses take from an inner wall of a living human cell as they are leaving it. This membrane not only gives the virus the ability to infect other cells, but because it contains fat, it is easily destroyed by chemicals such as ether or alcohol. These dissolve the fat, thereby killing the virus. The only cells that herpes simplex and zoster can infect other than in laboratory experiments are human cells. Humans, therefore, are the only carriers of these germs and the only ones who can pass it on. It is not possible for you to contract either simplex or zoster from an animal such as a dog or cat.

It has also recently been found that these viruses, as well as CMV and Epstein-Barr (E-B) virus, share not only a similar physical appearance and certain disease characteristics, but the all-crucial ability to infect our bodies chronically and forever by traveling to certain of our tissues during our first infection. Work by such researchers as Stephens, Cook, and Baringer showed that once there they "set up shop" and lived quietly in what is called a latent state (see "Latency and Reactivation of Disease"), able at any time to cause a new attack of painful disease. Much of our present research into treatment of herpes is now aimed at killing or at least blocking release of infectious virus from these tissues. As we shall discuss later, we have high hopes in this area today.

Life Cycle of the Herpes Viruses

The first event to take place when the herpes virus infects a cell is the adsorption or sticking of the virus to the cell's outer membrane. Due to the action of special enzymes from the cell itself, the virus rapidly penetrates through the membrane and gains access to the cytoplasm inside the cell. Once inside, the cell continues to cooperate in its own future destruction by releasing enzymes which strip the fatty membrane from the virus and free the herpetic genetic material, the chromosome, still enclosed in its protein coat. This naked virus capsid is then carried to the cell's nucleus, the location of the cell's own genetic material and site from which most cellular manufacturing operations are directed. Once in the nucleus, the viral chromosome (which is called DNA) is released and takes over directing all cellular activity. The cell and all its components go to work producing new viral components under the direction of the invading viral genetic DNA. New herpes DNA is manufactured in the nucleus and new protein coats are manufactured in the cytoplasm. The protein coats travel into the nucleus, where they merge with the viral DNA to form new, noninfectious, naked capsids.

The number of viruses produced by each cell in this manner is most impressive. It is estimated that between 80,000–120,000 new herpes viruses are manufactured by each infected cell. The entire process takes only three to five hours from the time of penetration of the infecting single virus. Once the naked capsids have been formed, they start their migration through the cell. As they pass through the cell membrane, they pick up a third coating from the cell wall itself. It is the addition of this third coating which makes the new herpes viruses infectious. The cell wall then ruptures to release thousands upon thousands of new infectious organisms into the bloodstream or surrounding tissues, where they are then free to infect yet further cells. One would think that the production of so many thousands of viruses so rapidly would cause an overwhelming infection in any one of us. Fortunately, our bodies are quite capable of handling almost all herpes infections quite safely, using our own immune systems which are made up of white blood cells and antibodies in the blood. Our body defenses against herpes will be discussed in more detail later.

All of the invading herpes viruses do not cause an active infection of the cells resulting in production of new virus and death of the invaded cell. Some of the viruses will enter the latent stage. Our present understanding of latency indicates that the invading virus does penetrate the cell and is uncoated in the cytoplasm. The viral DNA then either makes its way to the nucleus or may possibly remain in the cytoplasm in a nonactive state. It may remain in this quiet state living as a harmless inhabitant of the cell until such a time as a stressful inciting factor activates the viral chromosomes and causes them to go into a reproductive state which results in the production of new virus and the death of the host cell.

All herpes viruses reproduce in much the same way that herpes simplex does; they replicate and rupture the cells to be released into the surrounding tissue. Herpes zoster, however, is rarely if ever released from the cell completely. Rather, this virus tends to cling to or become part of the cell wall and is, therefore, separated only with great difficulty from the membrane involved in the infected tissue. Nonetheless, zoster virus infection of cells can be and is as highly destructive as any other herpes infection.

Herpes Infection: Common to Every Social and Economic Class?

But who exactly gets herpes infection? Is it more confined to one social or income group than another or is it an infection which attacks all classes and races with equal frequency? With zoster, the first attack is chicken pox—and almost always quite noticeable. It infects all classes and races equally. In the case of herpes simplex, the answers to these questions have changed radically within the last forty years.

In the earliest studies done during the 1940s, there were, of course, only two populations to be studied: those people who had herpetic antibodies in their blood and those who didn't. There was no subdivision into those who had genital herpes and those who had oral herpes. The early studies found a relatively low (40 percent) incidence of herpes antibodies among medical students who were considered representative of the "solid middle class."[6] In contrast, more than 90 percent of the hospital ward patients from low-income areas had evidence of herpetic infection. In similar studies done during the 1960s, private patients in hospitals were found to have only about 60 percent evidence of herpes infection, while nearly 85 percent of the ward patients of low income had evidence of infection.[26] Similarly, only 30 percent of college students and young doctors studied during this period had had herpes infections. Twenty years ago, then, infection among the upper social classes tended to occur after early childhood and, in some groups studied, only 40 percent of the adults had evidence of ever being infected by herpes. Almost all patients in these studies were white, however.

Other studies were done to see if there was a difference in the frequency of herpes infections among whites and blacks. In a South African study, it was found that the white population had a very low incidence of herpes infection, while blacks living in the city had a high incidence of herpes infection. The highest incidence of herpes infection of all, however, was found among the Bantus, a tribe of very poor blacks living in close, unclean rural quarters.[3]

As in the African study, the effect of poor housing and crowded conditions on a person's chance of contracting herpes was shown in an English study, where a decrease in the frequency of herpes infection was demonstrated after a large population of people were moved into better housing conditions and given better facilities for good hygiene.[42]

These older studies, then, showed that if you were poor or black or lived in crowded or unclean conditions, you had a much greater chance of become infected with herpes simplex virus. But

Table II: Herpes Simplex Virus Disease Survey Research Project

Purpose: To collect demographic, socioeconomic, medical, attitudinal, and behavioral information about the magnitude, severity, and impact of herpes simplex virus disease on the lives of patients.

Method:	Six-Page Mail Questionnaire					
	No. Sent	No. Returned	Excluded (diagnosis uncertain)			Total
	7,500	3,780 (50.40)	638 (16.88)			3,142

Summary Results (percent of total)

Sex:	Men	Women				
	48.85	51.15				

Age:	Mean	0–14 yrs.	15–19 yrs.	20–24 yrs.	25–29 yrs.	30–34 yrs.	35–39 yrs.	Over 40
	33.3 yrs	0.06	0.73	11.39	29.98	26.10	12.73	19.04

Ethnicity:	Caucasian	Black	Hispanic	Oriental	Native American	Other
	95.12	1.59	1.18	0.25	1.46	0.38

Marital Status:	Married	Separated	Divorced	Widow/Widower	Single
	36.05	2.77	21.94	1.43	37.80

Annual Earnings:	0–5K	5–10K	10–15K	15–20K	20–25K	26–35K	36–45K	Over 46K	Unknown
	4.71	8.34	14.86	15.60	12.13	18.90	9.46	13.21	2.80

School Yrs. Compl.:	01–11 yrs.	12 yrs.	13–15 yrs.	16 yrs.	17–18 yrs.	19–20 yrs.	21+ yrs.
	2.20	19.35	25.14	28.04	16.14	7.03	1.91

Sexual Preference:	Heterosexual	Homosexual	Bisexual
	94.34	2.64	3.02

Prob. Source of Infection:	Unknown	Spouse	Steady	Casual	Rape
	20.82	9.85	34.04	34.14	1.16

Time:*	1–3 mos.	4–6 mos.	7–11 mos.	1–3 yrs.	Over 4 yrs.
	70.05	9.69	7.63	7.44	5.19

Money Spent on Rx and/or Treatment and Remedies:	None	$1–50	$51–100	$101–250	$251–750	$751–1,500	$1,501–3,000	Over $3,001
	7.09	27.00	21.45	22.25	13.88	4.27	2.30	1.31

Total Known Individuals Infected by Respondents: 2,023 infected by 1,120 respondents; 2,103 indicated no known spread

* Length of time from the perception of illness until diagnosis medically established

* Knox, S., Corey, L., Blough, H., Lerner, M. "Historical Findings in Subjects from a High Socioeconomic Group Who Have Genital Infections with Herpes Simplex," *Sexually Transmitted Diseases*, 9:15, 1982. With permission

social patterns have changed in the last two decades and herpes simplex has achieved a new status in our lives. As we have found greater freedom in our living patterns and the variety in sexual activity has increased among all classes of people, we can now find far fewer differences among those who have herpes infections and those people who do not. The chances of acquiring such an infection appear to be rising equally in all groups across the board.

The results of many studies now indicate that during the first four years of life there is a rapid rise in the rate of *nonvenereal* herpes simplex type-1 infections. About 70 percent of fourteen-year-olds have type-1 virus latent in their bodies. The virus is usually *caught silently by contact with a relative or friend with an unnoticed cold sore.* This does not mean that we should avoid relatives and friends. On the contrary, *this is how we normally get our initial herpes infections, infections which 95 percent of the time cause no obvious illness the first time around* and which may later provide partial protection from another strain of herpes. In the early teens, we also begin to see the appearance of and rise in infections with herpes simplex type-2. This, of course, coincides with the start of sexual activity among these young people. On the average, one out of every three thirty-five-year-olds has type-2 infection, and by age fifty years nine out of every ten Americans have either or both type-1 and type-2 herpes simplex virus residing in their bodies.

In a recent study on the social and economic background of a large group of people with genital herpes infections, we learned a number of previously unknown facts as shown in Table II.[28] This was a study of more than three thousand men and women from the middle to high social and economic classes. All of these people had recurring genital herpes. They were a highly motivated group and members of the national herpes organization, HELP, a division of the American Social Health Association in Palo Alto, California. The average age of the people involved in this study was thirty-three years and 95 percent of them were white. Approximately one third were married, one third single, and one third separated or divorced. Seventy-seven percent of these people had completed three years of college and 53 percent had college degrees. Their income level was also in the middle- and upper-middle-class range, with 55 percent of these people earning more than $20,000 annually and 70 percent earning more than $15,000.

Probable sources of infection were a steady boyfriend or girlfriend in one third of the cases, a casual sexual encounter in another third, from a spouse only 10 percent of the time, and unknown 20 percent of the time. Three women acquired their infections after being raped. Women tended to become infected earlier than the men (twenty-six versus thirty years), but both groups had had their infections an average of three and a half to four years.

In men, the penis was the area most commonly involved in first infections; in women, it was the external genitalia (vulva). Recurrences occurred at a rate of five to eight attacks yearly, with nearly half these people reporting that their attacks became less frequent with the passage of time. Only one out of five felt their recurrences were increasing in number. When the recurrent infections came, they appeared on the penis, vulva, mouth, face, rectum, buttocks, thighs, and/or abdomen.

You may or may not be discouraged by the recurrence rates in this group of patients. In general, they should be encouraging; nearly half of these people felt their disease course was improving. In addition, you should remember that the members of this group were all from a self-help group made up of people who, in the beginning, were having difficulty with their herpetic infection. We do not yet know how many millions of Americans have genital herpes just once or a few times and then have no further problems with it. They would not feel the need to join a support group; their data, therefore, could not be included in this study. If we could know those figures, they might well serve to make what information we have even more encouraging.

Other interesting information which was learned from this study involved treatment cost and spread of disease to sexual partners. Of the three thousand or so people involved, two out of three had spent less than $250 on either diagnostic or therapeutic remedies, while nine people had spent between $1,500 and $3,000. Two out of every three members of this group had continued to have sexual activity and indicated that, to their knowledge, they had not spread their infection to any sexual partner.

The remaining one thousand plus patients reported, however, that they had infected just over two thousand sexual contacts since becoming infected with their own illness. We do not know, however, what, if any, precautions these people or their sexual partners had taken to protect the uninfected person from contracting the herpetic infection. Perhaps one of the most important factors to come out of this study on genital herpes, then, is that it is an illness which now crosses all social and economic barriers and is one from which no one is immune.

Latency and Reactivation of Disease

We have already touched upon latency in our discussion of the "Life Cycle of the Herpes Viruses." During your first infection, various herpes viruses have various ways of establishing themselves chronically in your body. Herpes simplex type-1 travels from your skin or mouth, through the nerves, to your deep nerve centers (ganglia) near the brain and upper spinal cord. Herpes type-2 goes to the ganglia at the base of your spinal cord near your buttocks. Herpes zoster probably also infects the spinal nerve ganglia, but this has not yet been proven conclusively. CMV (cytomegalovirus) persistently infects cells in your kidneys, urinary, and genital system, as well as certain critical white blood cells known as B-lymphocytes and neutrophils. These cells are very important in fighting off infections of all kinds. As you will see in "The Gay Population and Herpetic Infections," interference with these white cells can result in a devastating illness. The E-B virus, the mononucleosis virus, apparently infects only the B-lymphocytes, but even this causes a drawn-out, fatiguing disease, and in Africans it causes cancer. Once in their respective favored locations, these viruses usually go into a silent period of sleep called latency. If you are fortunate, the virus will never awaken again to cause further problems. In many cases of herpes simplex, unfortunately, the virus will reactivate, travel back down a few select nerves, and cause a blistering rash or eruption in the area fed by those nerves.

Factors which may cause reactivation of herpes simplex are all various forms of stress. These may but do not always include fever (fever blisters), a bad sunburn (sun blisters), physical exhaustion, emotional upsets, pregnancy, menstruation, masturbation, nonspecific irritation of the genitals (e.g., tight pants), and sexual intercourse. People who constantly get simplex blisters can often identify the factor or factors which reactivate their virus and take steps to avoid that form of stress. Examples of this would be taking aspirin to prevent fever at the first sign of the flu or being careful to tan slowly during the summer, rather than getting a "good burn" all in one day.

The cause of reactivation of zoster virus and the other human herpes viruses is not really known. Stress and chronic illness (such as eczema, poor nutrition, cancer, or drugs used to prevent rejection of organ transplants) appear to be involved. If you do not have a persistently debilitating illness, these are almost always once-in-a-lifetime attacks. Therefore, you do not often get a chance to identify other specific factors which may cause these diseases to become active.

Body Defenses Against Infection by Herpes Viruses

Usually when you are infected by a virus or bacteria, your body produces special blood plasma proteins (called antibodies) and special white blood cells (helper and suppressor lymphocytes, natural killer cells, macrophages) which kill the germs. Both systems, antibody and white cell, usually last for years or even a lifetime, thus protecting you from being reinfected by the same germs. The herpes viruses are no different in stimulating your body to produce antiviral antibodies and cells. They are different from most other germs, however, in that they are protected from the killer action of these systems by staying safely inside your body's cell walls where they cannot be reached. These viruses rarely enter the bloodstream again. They simply travel from one cell to its immediate neighbor by passing through walls that touch each other; they never expose themselves to the surrounding antibody containing tissue fluids or white cells. This is why someone who has perfectly good antiherpes antibodies and white cells can still get one herpes attack after another simply from reactivation of the latent virus already in the nerve cells.

Perhaps more discouraging is the fact that infection with one herpes virus does not completely protect you from catching a second type of herpes virus. There are several cases of patients who have had many cold sores from herpes simplex type-1 catching another strain of type-1 in the eye or type-2 in the genital area. As a rule, however, these second infections are not as severe as first infection, which caused visibly apparent diseases. This indicates that there is at least partial protection from the antibodies and white cells stimulated by the first herpes infection. In the case of zoster, most infections are thought to be reactivations of chicken pox virus latent in a nerve ganglion. There are reports, however, of people coming down with "shingles" after being exposed to someone with chicken pox or even to another person with "shingles."

4. GENITAL INFECTIONS

An Epidemic in the Making

Gonorrhea (clap) and syphilis have long been considered the two major sexually transmitted diseases. On February 20, 1979, however, a news release from the United Press International (UPI) described an organization called HELP, Herpetics Engaged in Living Productively. HELP was founded by the American Social Health Association to call attention to and to assist the then estimated five to twenty million Americans affected by a major health problem, genital herpes, a problem which they, and often their doctors, did not understand. Certainly, untreated genital herpes infection does not constitute quite the same threat to you as does untreated syphilis or gonorrhea. In a very short period of time, gonorrhea can cause such severe inflammation in the womb as to cause permanent sterility; over a several-year period, syphilis can cause insanity, blindness, paralysis, and death. But syphilis and gonorrhea can be permanently cured with common antibiotics and, as yet, genital herpes can not. With several million people already infected with genital herpes and the number climbing every day, venereal herpes is passing all other sexually contracted diseases in sheer numbers. It has reached epidemic proportions with five hundred thousand new cases contracted each year.

Herpes-2 is the most common cause of genital sores in women and is second only to syphilis in men.

Because of the way it is spread, we rarely see genital herpes in young children. But by the early teen years, as sexual contact begins, the incidence of infection has been shown to rise abruptly and continue to rise for the next twenty years. As we have also noted, herpes formerly was a disease found more commonly among people with lower incomes and those living in poor and crowded conditions. In the past ten years, however, the liberation movements have introduced a new and widespread sexual freedom which has allowed herpes widespread access to the very highest social and income levels. Genital herpes has now established itself in the most inner circles of wealth and power.

How the Infection Is Passed On

Herpes has been nicknamed the "virus of love" because the mode of spread is usually by intimate body contact, whether by kissing or sexual intercourse. Sexual spread may be by as many routes as one can devise for lovemaking: genital-to-genital, mouth-to-genital, genital-to-mouth, rectal-to-genital, and mouth-to-rectum. Although we commonly associate herpes type-2 with a genital location, it is not surprising to find herpes type-1 in the genitalia of patients who practice cunnilingus (contact with the female genitalia by mouth) or herpes type-2 in the throats of patients who perform fellatio (penis taken into the mouth). Such a patient case is discussed under "Venereal Herpes Outside the Genital Area." The changing frequency with which we find type-1 herpes in the genital area and type-2 around the face and mouth is an interesting indicator of our recent changes in sexual behavior. Twenty years ago, only one in twenty patients with venereally acquired herpes had type-2 "above the waist" and type-1 "below the waist." This meant there was little mouth-to-genital sex play. Within ten years, however, these figures had climbed to nearly four out of every twenty such patients having type-2 in the mouth and type-1 in the genitalia. Not surprisingly, the greatest increase in type-1 herpes infections of the genitals occurred in the fifteen- to twenty-four-year-old age group. One out of three people with venereal herpes under the age of twenty-four years had type-1 genital disease, while only seven out of one hundred people over the age of twenty-five years had venereal type-1.[15] The sexual revolution of the 1960s clearly mixed up the usual site-specificity of types 1 and 2 because of the great increase in oral-genital contact. Masturbation or nonsexual close body contact, as in wrestling (*Herpes gladiatorum*) or rugby (*Herpes rugbeiform*), are also excellent ways of spreading virus from a genital or nongenital site to almost any other location in the body (see "Athletics and Herpes").

It should also be remembered that venereal herpes is frequently associated with and may initially be hidden by other forms of genital infection. These include not just syphilis and gonorrhea but fungal infection, Trichomonas, bacterial vaginitis, and venereal warts, any of which must be treated and cured before the full extent of genital herpes may be appreciated or perhaps even diagnosed. Indeed, the study discussed previously under "Herpes Infection: Common to Every Social and Economic Class?" reported that, of more than three thousand genital herpes patients questioned, nearly two out of ten had had gonorrhea or NGU (a venereal disease called nongonorrheal urethritis) and nearly six out of ten had had syphilis!

The Nature of First Infection (Primary Infection)

The first infection with herpes usually occurs three to seven days after sexual exposure. Many people never notice this first attack, indicating that it may be quite mild, with just a few tiny blisters or even totally without signs or symptoms. As mentioned, patients who have had previous infection with type-1 virus, such as a cold sore on the mouth, usually have some partial protection against severe infection with herpes type-2. If there is a question in your mind as to whether you have recently had genital herpes, your doctor can draw two blood tests for herpes antibodies, usually one month apart (acute and long-term levels). Even if you just want to know if you have ever had either type, these tests are often very useful, although a distinction between the two types cannot always be made because of cross-reaction between the antibodies.

In those several hundred thousand people who do develop active disease each year, the symptoms of mild tingling and burning may precede the actual appearance of lesions. Within a matter of hours, watery blisters will develop. Herpes virus is *most infectious during the blistering stage,* least infectious during the crusted stage, *but may even be passed on to someone else during the tingling stage just before the appearance of any blisters.*

In women, these blisters are often extensive, involving the external genitalia (the labia, perirectal skin, foreskin of the clitoris), as well as the vagina and cervix, which protrudes into the vaginal canal from the end of the womb (uterus). There is often much watery discharge and pain on urination.

In men, groups of blisters appear on the head, foreskin, or shaft of the penis. In the past, these have sometimes been confused with syphilitic ulcers. Acute herpes of the penis may produce tremendous painful swelling of the organ and leave the patient with narrowing of the urinary opening such that he has subsequent difficulty "passing water" and must undergo dilation therapy even after the acute disease has passed.

In both men and women, there may be associated low-grade fever, headache, generalized muscle aching, and tender, swollen lymph nodes in the groin. Twenty-four to forty-eight hours after their appearance, the blisters break down to leave raw red areas of ulceration which form grayish membranes and then crust over, dry, and heal without treatment and without scarring. The entire course of a florid first infection lasts three to six weeks. The following is a case report of a young man with an unusually severe primary herpes infection involving not only his genitalia but spread to several other areas of his body. Despite the severity of his primary infection, he made a most successful long-term recovery.[35]

A thirty-seven-year-old white man was first seen complaining of pain in his penis and groin, discomfort and difficulty with urination, and a slight discharge from his penis for the past two days. These symptoms had developed about five days after having sexual intercourse with a stranger. Examination revealed that he had a bloodstained discharge from his penis and that the end of his penis was very inflamed. A diagnosis of nonspecific infection of the penile urinary tract was made and he was treated with antibacterial drugs. He returned four days later, much more ill and complaining of difficulty breathing, dizziness, and confusion. He was admitted to the hospital. Examination revealed a blackened area of skin surrounding the end of his penis and flattened pustules in the area of badly damaged tissue. The entire penis was swollen, hot, and reddened. Dome-shaped cloudy blisters of varying sizes were spread widely over the skin of his scalp, neck, chin, trunk, buttocks, scrotum, fingers, shoulders, thighs, and feet. He had a high fever, looked very ill, and was drowsy and confused. A series of sophisticated electronic and X-ray tests of his brain function fortunately revealed no other abnormalities.

Virus cultures were taken from several of the sores scattered across his body and all grew out herpes simplex type-2. Blood tests for antibodies also indicated that this was a primary infection with type-2 herpes. There was also no evidence on blood-testing that he had had previous infection with type-1 herpes and, therefore, had no cross-protection against type-2 infection.

The patient was still treated with antibiotics to protect him against any undetected bacterial infection which might be present. The sores on his penis and all other herpes lesions scattered across his body were opened and cleaned out before being painted with a 5 percent solution of the antiviral idoxuridine (IDU) in DMSO (dimethyl sulfoxide).* This procedure was carried out three times daily for five days and was followed by rapid improvement. The pustules healed and there was a minimal loss of tissue from the end of his penis. He was discharged after one week in the hospital.

When he was seen again one week later, narrowing of his urinary canal from scars was treated by dilation.

He remained well for the ensuing nine months, at which time he developed a cluster of herpes type-2 blisters on his right heel. These healed within a few days but returned again one month later with similar blisters on his left foot, neck,

---

* Not FDA-approved for drug use in the United States.

stomach, and left ring finger; all were sites of blisters during his first illness. Herpes type-2 was cultured from these recurrent sores.

In the three years of follow-up since that time, the patient has remained well and has had no noticeable recurrent herpes.

While this young man had an unusually severe first attack of genital herpes, it is quite typical of what we expect to see in patients, male or female, who have not been infected previously with either herpes simplex type-1 or type-2. This young man was in otherwise perfect health and yet he had no blood antibodies or white cells which were immediately available to fight and control spread of the herpes infection from his genital area. Nonetheless, because of his basic good health his body was able to muster an appropriate response to successfully heal all disease.

The apparent dramatic response to the antiviral drug IDU in DMSO is difficult to evaluate because of the variability in healing time from patient to patient. We can not, therefore, conclude from this single case study that this therapy increased the speed of recovery from his primary illness. We can conclude, however, that it did nothing to prevent recurrent attacks in later months. Perhaps the most encouraging note is the observation that after several attacks within the first few months of his illness, he had no further difficulties with his disease.

Frequency of Recurrent Attacks

Fortunately, not every patient who has had an episode of genital herpes will necessarily develop recurrent infections. Many will never have obvious disease again, while others will go into extended periods of chronic, repeated episodes of active ulceration for months or years. Many patients report that the disease then quiets down spontaneously, for reasons which are not understood. More studies proving this are yet to be published, however. It seems encouraging to know that as time passes, attacks will come farther and farther apart and each successive one will be a bit less severe than the one which preceded it. Further medical research will answer this definitively for us.

The chances of another attack vary from study to study, but in general, five to eight out of every ten people who have had an attack of primary genital herpes will suffer a recurrent infection within three months of the first episode. Additionally, *if your genital infection is herpes type-1, you have about five times less chance of recurrent infection than if your genital infection is due to type-2.*[37] In this sense, then, oral-genital sex may be preferable to genital-genital sex. If you do have a type-2 infection, your chances of recurrence are less, however, if you develop high levels of blood antibody against this strain; in other words, if your body musters a very strong blood reaction against the virus.

There is some recent indication that the frequency of these attacks is related not only to the general health of the patient (chronically ill or stressed patients have more attacks) but to the virus strain itself. Some strains of virus are more prone to frequent reactivation and others tend to remain quietly latent in the body. The overwhelming majority of recurrent attacks, when they do occur, come from spontaneous reactivation of the latent virus in the deep nerve cells near the base of the spinal cord and rarely from exposure to new virus during sexual intercourse. If you have type-2 herpes in your genital nerve cells (ganglia), it will not protect you from catching type-1 through oral-genital contact or even from catching another strain of type-2. What pre-existing herpes type-1 or -2 infection anyplace in your body will do, however, is make the illness caused by a new virus much less severe than a true primary—first herpes ever—infection. This is because you will already have protective antibodies against herpes from the first herpes infection. Because the new virus infection is less severe than a rampant primary infection, it is often difficult for your doctor to tell if the blisters are due to reactivation of the old herpes you already have latent in your nerve ganglia or due to a new herpes virus picked up from someone else. Unless you have had sexual activity recently with someone with active herpes, the odds are strongly in favor of your new blisters simply being due to a recurrence of your own original herpes virus.

Causes of Recurrent Genital Infection

Precipitating factors have already been discussed, but include the usual stressful situations such as menstruation, emotional upset, pregnancy, and local trauma to the genitalia. Unlike type-1 herpes, however, fever does not seem to be an important activating factor for type-2 herpes. This is possibly because the virus is more easily damaged by heat, rather than stimulated by it. One need not have sexual intercourse to have a recurrent attack of herpes, but most people do report having had sexual activity within ten days of onset of their illness.

Nature of Recurring Infections

Recurrent blisters and ulcers may frequently be inconspicuous and not noticed on casual inspection, but they are contagious to any partner in sexual activity. Occasionally, women may have active but "invisible" infection, as they may develop their recurrent blisters—only deep inside the vaginal canal on the cervix; men may have live virus in the semen but no penile sores. There may be no symptoms and, being unaware of the reactivation of their virus, they may not warn a sexual partner to take precautions (see "Silent Infections"). The genital sites involved when blisters do appear are the same as those seen in first infections, but are always (in a healthy patient) smaller localized patches of blisters which break within forty-eight hours to leave red shallow ulcers. Other sites frequently involved in recurrent disease are the rectum, buttocks, thighs, abdomen, and mouth. The combination of genital and urinary tract herpes infection is much more common in postmenopausal than in premenopausal women. These may cause local pain and burning on urination, but there is very rarely fever, headache, or other symptomatology such as is found with the initial attack. Healing is more rapid than in initial infections and takes place within seven to ten days, leaving the involved surfaces normal and totally without scarring. During recurrent attacks, you are contagious from about one day before the blisters appear until scabbing has taken place (about three to six days).

Silent Infections

Perhaps the greatest contributing factor to spread of herpetic venereal disease is the silent but contagious state of infection in both men and women. Some men and women may shed live infectious virus from their genitalia without ever having developed noticeable evidence of disease. Even a careful examination by a physician will fail to reveal blisters or ulcers, but virus cultures or Pap smears are almost invariably diagnostically positive. Women may shed from the external genital lips or from inside the vaginal canal and the cervix. Men may shed from anywhere on the penis or in the semen during ejaculation.

The frequency with which herpes virus is isolated from previously infected women who have no current signs of disease varies from one to ten of every one hundred women. The following are case examples taken from one study on five women with a history of genital herpes.[1] All women were found to have positive virus cultures intermittently for weeks to months after all signs of infection had cleared. These five cases are presented as examples of recurrent shedding of live virus from the genitalia during periods when doctors could find no physical signs of herpes and the women were feeling entirely well. The social and sexual history of these women is presented in Table III.

Patient 1: A twenty-eight-year-old woman developed primary genital herpes, from which type-2 virus was cultured. Seven days later, examination showed that the lesions were healing, but virus was still present in the external genitalia and in the cervix. Two weeks later, there was no sign of disease anywhere, but virus was still cultured from the cervix within the vaginal canal. Five weeks later, the patient was feeling entirely well, there was no sign of any disease on medical examination, yet herpes virus type-2 was still recovered from cervical cultures.

Patient 2: This twenty-five-year-old woman was found to have recurrent herpes of her genitalia. However, virus cultures taken from ulcers on the external genitalia and the cer-

Table III: Social and Sexual History of Five Women Who Shed Herpes-2 from Their Genitalia Without Evidence of Clinical Disease

	Patient 1	Patient 2	Patient 3	Patient 4	Patient 5
Age	28	25	25	23	21
Education	High School	College (4 yrs.)	College and Grad School	College	College (3 yrs.)
Marital Status	Divorced	Married	Single	Divorced	Single
Pregnancies?	0	0	0	1	0
Age at First Intercourse	19	21	21	20	20
Age at First Pregnancy	—	—	—	20	—
Total No. of Sex Partners During Lifetime	30	6	10	6	20
Oral-Genital Contact	Yes	Yes	Yes	Yes	Yes
Other VD	No	No	No	No	No
History of Oral Herpes	Yes	No	No	No	No
Type of Contraceptive Used	Oral*	Oral*	Oral*	Oral*	IUD†

* On oral contraceptive at time of symptomatic genital herpes
† IUD = intrauterine device
* Adapted from: Adam, E., Kaufman, R., Mirkovic, R., Melnick, J. "Persistence of Virus Shedding in Asymptomatic Women After Recovery from Herpes Genitalis." Reprinted with permission from the American College of Obstetricians and Gynecologists, *Obstetrics and Gynecology* 54:173, 1979.

vix, both on the first and eighth day of examination, grew out no herpes. This young woman was feeling totally well when seen six weeks and eleven weeks after her first examination and, although no virus could be cultured from her genitals on the six-week examination, she was found to be shedding live, infectious virus on the eleven-week examination, despite the absence of any signs of disease.

Patient 3: This twenty-five-year-old woman also had recurrent genital herpes with cultures positive for type-2. When she was examined five days later, there was no sign of any disease involving her genitalia and her virus cultures were negative. She was seen again three and five weeks later, at which time she was feeling entirely well and had no signs of herpetic disease. Nonetheless, herpes type-2 was cultured from the cervix during an exam on the seventh week.

Patient 4: This twenty-three-year-old woman suffered a recurrent attack of genital herpes, yet cultures for virus taken on day four and seven, when the lesions appeared healed, were negative. However, when she came for follow-up examination, nearly ten months later, no evidence of herpetic disease was present on examination, but cultures of her cervix revealed that she was shedding live herpes virus type-2.

Patient 5: A twenty-one-year-old woman developed primary genital herpes, from which type-2 virus was cultured. Ten days later, her disease had healed completely, but virus was still isolated from her cervix. One month later, she was feeling entirely well and her cultures for virus were negative. Two and one-half months after her initial attacks of herpes, she had recurrent genital infection with positive virus isolation. Two months after her recurrence, she was entirely well and no virus could be cultured from her genitalia. However, four months after her recurrent attack, she was seen because of discomfort from her intrauterine contraceptive device. There was no evidence of herpetic sores anywhere on the genitalia, yet herpes type-2 was cultured from her cervix.

Perhaps the main lesson we might learn from the above cases is that, like men, it is very difficult for women to tell when they are, in fact, capable of infecting their sexual partners. None of the women described above developed any notable genital herpetic disease within three weeks after live virus had been isolated from their genitalia. Neither were any of these women aware of obvious genital herpes in their recent sex partners at the time virus was isolated from them while they appeared free of disease. This indicates that it is unlikely that their positive cultures came from recent sexual activity with an infected partner, but it can not be completely discounted either.

The questions that are useful to ask yourself as a woman who may have genital herpes are: 1) are there certain periods of your life that you can identify as times when you are likely to shed virus—for instance, during your premenstrual period; 2) is your virus-shedding related to certain conditions, such as stress, emotional upset, or physical exhaustion; 3) could your virus-shedding be related to the type of contraception you use—i.e., is an intrauterine device more likely to stir up the virus than oral contraceptives or mechanical forms of contraception such as diaphragms and condoms; 4) and last, but worth at least some consideration, is the amount of virus you shed really sufficient to spread the infection? The answers to the first three questions you will work out over time. As you get your Pap smears done by your gynecologist every six months, try to correlate what was going on in your life around the time that any one or more smears was reported positive for herpes. A pattern to guide you as to when sexual activity is safe will usually develop. The answer to the fourth question is not yet known. We have not yet established the minimum amount or the virulence of virus necessary to allow the spread of infection from a herpes carrier to someone who does not yet have the illness.

An even greater number of men than women may serve as unrecognized sources of genital herpes infection in their sex partners. It has been shown in one study that infectious herpes virus can be recovered from prostatic and vas deferens fluid in nearly fifteen out of every one hundred male patients who have absolutely no history of genital herpes infection.[11] Shedding of live virus from men who have had known genital herpes in the past

obviously would be much higher (asymptomatic). Men should
also ask themselves some of the questions just suggested for
women. You too may be silent shedders and, while you may
not have the advantage of the Pap smears to guide you, you can
certainly use condoms and contraceptive (viricidal) gels during
any times of doubt.

Rectal Infection

Rectal herpes (proctitis) may develop after either heterosexual
(opposite sex) or homosexual (same sex) anal intercourse. Although we do not know the exact incidence of rectal infection
with herpes virus, the increasing number of men who engage in
homosexual or bisexual activity and women who engage in sodomy (anal intercourse) would make us conclude that the incidence of herpes infections around the rectum is increasing
steadily. Almost every case of rectal herpes is the result of anal
intercourse. However, some men and women who have been infected with genital herpes may have a spontaneous spread of their
ulcers to the rectal area from their external genitalia. Because of
the way rectal herpes is acquired, the viral type which causes it is
usually herpes type-2. We should remember, however, that anal
herpes can be contracted from oral-anal contact with a sexual
partner who has a cold sore on his or her mouth. In these cases,
the virus type recovered on culture is herpes type-1, but the disease resulting from type-1 is not significantly different from that
caused by herpes-2.

The infection itself is severely painful and may be the most
common cause of acute inability to urinate. The active disease
develops within ten days of exposure and presents as raw ulceration of the mucous membrane around the anal opening and up the
rectal canal for about one and a half inches. From this point, ulcers do not develop, but local redness and occasional areas of
bleeding under the rectal surface tissues appear. The disease goes
away by itself in ten days to six weeks, depending on whether it is
a recurrent or first attack.

There is very little written in the medical literature about anal
herpes, but one study of eighteen patients with this illness may

give you some insight as to its nature.[23] Of the eighteen patients studied, sixteen were men and two were female. Fifteen of the men were homosexual and the sixteenth bisexual. The two women, neither of whom were married, engaged in sodomy, in addition to usual heterosexual intercourse. The age range of these patients was eighteen to forty years and, for an average of nine days before diagnosis was made, almost every patient had severe rectal pain. Other signs and symptoms included rectal itching, discharge, fever, chills, and feelings of being generally unwell. No patient had had any previous rectal or similar problem, although six had had rectal gonorrhea in the past. Two of the patients in this study had been incorrectly diagnosed elsewhere as having rectal gonorrhea during their present illness but had not responded to the usual antibiotic treatment.

On examination, the men and women in this study all had small blisters or ulcers on the skin around the anal opening and in the anal canal. Many of these patients had swollen glands in their groins as well. Herpes simplex virus was cultured from the lesions. Everyone recovered within three weeks of the onset of illness, with the average recovery time being eleven days. There were no recurrences of disease, with the exception of one patient who did develop recurrent herpes of the rectum nearly one year after his first attack.

The following is a case report typical of herpes virus type-2 infection of the anus.[10]

This twenty-nine-year-old man was admitted to the hospital because of five days of severe rectal pain, cramps, and diarrhea associated with fever, chills, and loss of appetite. The onset of his illness had been sudden with rectal discomfort, followed by watery diarrhea, a blood discharge, and pain in his lower abdomen. He had never had a similar illness and denied homosexual activity or contact with anyone else having a similar illness. He also denied ever having cold sores, a discharge from his penis, or ulcers.

Examination revealed an acutely ill young man who appeared quite pale. There was tenderness over the lower part of his abdomen, particularly on the left side. Groups of blisters surrounded the perianal area. Examination of the rectum revealed extreme tenderness and redness of the internal membrane for a distance of two inches up the rectal canal. There were also several small hemorrhages and ulcers in this area. The genital exam was normal and there were no swollen glands in his groin.

A diagnosis of herpes simplex proctitis was made.

No specific treatment was given and over the next few days, the patient began to feel generally better, although the rectal symptoms and ulcers remained. At the time of discharge ten days later, the sores were still present but improving. By twenty-one days after the onset of his illness, he was feeling entirely well and there was no sign of ulceration. He had no recurrences of his illness in the five months of follow-up.

For any of you who have experienced anal herpes, the disease can be most distressing indeed. The symptoms which precede the onset of the attack are usually mild, with simply local irritation, burning and numbness of the anal area. Within a short time, however, pain which may be excruciating and persistent will develop and last until the ulcers disappear. This pain may radiate to your groin, buttocks, and upper thighs. A watery discharge from the anal canal is common and may become purulent if bacterial infection enters the picture as well. An additional burden caused by herpes in the rectal canal is a reflex inhibition of moving your bowels. The trauma of stool passing over the ulcers in the anal canal can only serve to increase the pain and thus cause one to go to great lengths to avoid having a bowel movement.

While we know, then, that all patients with rectal herpes will recover within one to three weeks of the onset of their illness, the main problem of course is management of your acute illness during that time. It is important to reduce the irritation of the internal rectal ulcers by use of stool softeners and daily doses of bowel lubricants (such as mineral oil) taken orally as directed by your physician. These can greatly assist you in having a bowel movement which does not cause further irritation of the rectal ulcers. Equally important is your daily hygiene, which should involve twice-daily gentle washing of the area with a warm, mild, soapy solution, gentle rinsing, and very careful drying of the area.

Keeping the perirectal area dry is most important, as this will prevent further irritation of the ulcers and speed their healing.

As in genital infections, rectal herpes may also result in silent shedding of contagious live virus. Although it would not be obvious to a sexual partner, shedders may frequently be identified because of local redness of the rectal canal. This examination must be done by a physician, using a magnified view through a tube inserted into the rectum.

But while shedding of infectious herpes virus may occur without any obvious signs or symptoms of active infection and, therefore, must be a real concern both to the person who has such an anal infection and to his or her sexual partners, there is one area of concern that should be dismissed from your mind now. In recent years, we have all been concerned with an apparent connection between genital herpes and cervical or vulval cancer in women. Does such an association also exist in patients who have rectal infections? *As there has been no similar connection between herpes virus and cancer of the penis, it seems very unlikely that this viral infection would be associated with cancer of the anus or rectum.* Additionally, homosexuals who frequently practice anal intercourse have not been found to have a higher incidence of anal or rectal cancer than heterosexuals who do not engage in anal sexual practices.

Venereal Herpes Outside the Genital Area

Sexual foreplay and masturbation during periods of obvious or silent infections may result in spread of genital herpes, type-2 or -1, to a variety of other sites in the body. Ulcers may be found on the buttocks, the knees, back, lower abdomen, mouth, throat, and fingers.

Although we commonly think of herpes type-2 as involving the genital area and type-1 as confined to the mouth and eyes, the following is an example of type-2 infection located on an area of the body far from the genitalia.[24]

This young woman had had sexual relations with only one man for the past year. Her partner left town for a week and when he returned he noted a "bump" on his penis. The patient and her partner had intercourse on that day as well as oral-genital contact. Three days later, the patient noted an aching under her ears and one day after that, began to feel pain in her throat. Within twenty-four hours, she had developed pain in her external genitalia.

A medical examination two days later revealed a reddened throat and swollen glands in her neck. Examination of her genitalia revealed multiple shallow ulcers approaching the perianal area. There were also many ulcers with a shaggy exudate covering the cervix at the end of the vaginal canal. It was felt that this young woman had primary genital herpes infection. Her sexual partner was examined at that time and found to have crusted sores present on the back of the shaft of his penis.

The patient was seen again five days later, complaining of increased pain in her throat. Examination of this area revealed many shallow ulcers with a shaggy exudate in the back of her throat. No treatment was given but when seen again ten days later, she was feeling much improved and had several healing ulcers present on her external genitalia.

At this time, the results of virus cultures taken from her genitalia and throat on previous visits returned and were positive for herpes virus type-2. Herpes virus was not recovered from the crusted lesion of her male partner. However, blood tests for antibodies on both patients indicated that each one had recently become infected with herpes virus type-2.

The above case teaches us not only that genital herpes may grow anyplace in the body and recreate typical herpetic disease, but emphasizes the importance of avoiding sexual contact with your partner if there is any evidence of active herpetic infection. It would appear likely that the young man contracted herpes while he was on his out-of-town trip but had only a mild case of primary infection. Nonetheless, he was still infectious at the time he and this young woman had intercourse and oral-genital contact. Herpes type-2 was, therefore, passed onto her in both locations.

Of the other sites mentioned, red, swollen, watery *ulcers around the fingernails or on the fingers themselves* are a prime means for spreading disease, either through sexual or simply nonsexual contact. A good firm handshake may do to pass type-2 along. These lesions, known as "whitlows," are also a "red flag" to anyone who understands the nature of herpes. With the exception of people such as physicians, nurses, dentists, or oral hygienists, who may pick up either type-1 or type-2 herpes on their fingers from a patient with an infected mouth or genital area, whitlows often mean venereal disease. A bandage is a good solution to covering such a signal, as well as a means of preventing passing of the virus.

The following case report is typical of the excruciating discomfort which can be suffered by patients who have herpetic whitlows on their fingers. Although this is probably a type-1 infection, the illness produced by type-2 would be the same.[36]

> This patient was a thirty-eight-year-old dentist, who was seen for swelling, redness, severe pain and blister formation on his index finger. The surgeon initially diagnosed the problem as a bacterial infection and incised the area in an attempt to drain it. The cultures for bacteria were negative and there was no pus recovered from the infected site. The symptoms became more severe with increased pain, swelling and blistering of the end of the finger. Ultimately the dentist developed a fever and progressive inflammation of his right arm. He was admitted to hospital where virus studies revealed that the ulcers were due to a herpes virus infection of the finger, now also secondarily infected with bacteria. Treatment involved partial removal of the fingernail over the involved area and resulted in marked relief of pain by decompression of the blisters in the nailbed. Antibiotics were given for the accompanying bacterial infection and the dentist had fully recovered within twenty-one days.

The above case demonstrates how important differentiating a herpes infection from a bacterial infection of the finger can be. A misdiagnosis can only postpone the appropriate therapy and thereby prolong your pain and suffering.

Genital Herpes Without Sexual Contact

When many of us were children, our mothers warned us never to sit on public toilet seats for fear of catching some "dreadful" disease. For years, many public bathrooms had ultraviolet lights shining on the toilet seats in between use, as a means of sterilizing the surface and protecting users from disease. At that time there was, in fact, no real evidence that anyone caught any form of disease from a toilet seat. As years passed, many people ignored the warnings of their youth and did have direct contact with the seats in public bathrooms unless they were frankly wet and despite the fact that ultraviolet sterilization had long since been discontinued.

Now the possibility of catching a venereal disease from a toilet seat has raised its head again and this time with some scientific basis. It has been found that the herpes virus, which we previously believed died very quickly once exposed to a dry surface, is able to live up to four hours on a toilet seat—long enough to penetrate a small scratch in skin contacting the contaminated seat. Even more worrisome is the fact that these viruses may live as long as three days on cloth. Perhaps we need not be overly concerned with catching venereal disease from toilet seats, although this is not a ridiculous possibility. We should be concerned, however, with the fact that the virus does survive in cloth, and patients who have genital herpes should make every effort to use his or her own towels and facecloths during a recurrent episode and make sure that no one else uses any material with which the area of outbreak has been in contact. Equally important is remembering that active oral herpes virus can spread to a towel or facecloth through contact with a cold score during bathing and then to someone else's genitalia or face when that person rubs his own body with the same cloth. This is one obvious way of catching herpes type-1 in the genital region without sexual contact. If you do not have herpes, take the precaution of using your own toilet articles if someone else has a cold sore or is known to have any form of active herpes.

Diagnosis of Genital Herpes

The diagnosis of active genital herpes is highly accurate when based on the physical findings of genital blisters and ulcers alone. You should consult a physician at once if you suspect that you have the infection. Hospital emergency rooms are good places to go if your own doctor is not available. Your physician usually will be able to tell you whether or not you have genital herpes and, if he or she feels it is indicated, will take a Pap or Tzanck smear from your genital area for further proof of diagnosis. These are simple, painless tests which are particularly useful for detecting both active and silent infection. The smears often show the typical giant ballooning of the infected cells, thus indicating presence of herpes virus.

Other than the usual Pap or Tzanck smears, your doctor may also want to send a sample of your blood to the State Virology Laboratory to have antibody levels for herpes types 1 and 2 done at the time you are first examined and again a few weeks later. If the second sample shows a strong rise in antibody against one of the herpes viruses compared to the first blood sample, it means that the attack of blistering you have was due to that type of virus. It should be pointed out, however, that these blood tests are not 100 percent reliable if the levels of antibody in the two samples are low or the same, as there is some cross-reaction between the two virus types in antibody assays.

If your doctor is unsure or unable to make a definite diagnosis, you should be referred immediately to a specialist who is familiar with the infection. It is important for you to know whether you have genital herpes or not. In more highly specialized medical centers, such as at university hospitals, your doctor may not only take smears and blood tests but gently wipe your blisters with a cotton-tipped swab for a virus culture. Once the virus grows in the laboratory, it can be identified as herpes type-1 or -2.

5. PSYCHOLOGICAL ASPECTS OF HERPETIC ILLNESS

The Personal Effects of Recurrent Genital Herpes

It is difficult to understand the enormity of often unnecessary human suffering and personal tragedy which can be caused by herpes. The following are adaptations taken from just a few of thousands of letters and telephone calls I have received from patients with herpes. In some cases, these people had ruined personal lives, others knew little or nothing about their disease, a few had had a very dissatisfying relationship with a doctor, and still others had spent vast quantities of time and money on unsuccessful new treatment procedures. The *happiest* people were those who had found support groups made up of people with similar problems with herpes. The support groups provided sympathetic understanding, companionship, useful information, and a sense of purpose in life. But, most importantly, with time (usually two to three years), many members of these groups found that, having found new strength and courage within the group, they gradually became less dependent upon that support. They "outgrew" the herpes organizations and merged back into their former social groups with feelings of full confidence and acceptance.

Thirty-six-year-old male physician: "I am writing to find out if your new drug [Ara-AMP*] can help me. I caught herpes on my first date with a woman I hardly knew. For a year now, my attacks are so frequent it has been like getting a period every month. Now I know what women must feel like. It really ruins my social life. I'm divorced. Can I ever hope to marry again?"

Author's comment: While Ara-AMP appears to be too toxic for human use, broad therapeutic advances with drugs, such as acyclovir, are now being made as discussed later. As a study cited earlier has shown, this young physician should be encouraged by the finding that nearly half the genital herpes patients felt their illness was improving with time (fewer recurrences) and only one out of five felt it was worse.[28] As far as marriage is concerned, he should most certainly actively plan to marry again if he desires. This might best be done, however, after he has joined a herpes self-help group or entered short-term psychotherapy to regain self-esteem, companionship, and be brought up to date on new developments in the field. Self-help groups and psychotherapy are discussed in greater detail in "Regaining Your Self-Esteem and Social Life: Sources of Support and How They Work." When he ultimately meets a potential marriage partner, the support group

* Ara-AMP is Ara-A (vidarabine) with a phosphorus molecule attached.

or therapist may be of invaluable help to her in understanding herpes most sympathetically and supportively if she does not have genital herpes.

Fifty-six-year-old male newspaper magnate: "My doctor is treating me with dye-light therapy for herpes ulcers. Every day I lose two hours of valuable time painting my privates and sitting in front of a light bulb. This therapy has cost me almost $3,000. I'd pay even more for a better treatment than this. I don't believe it works."

Author's comment: Unfortunately, dye-light therapy has now been discredited as a useful means for combating either type-1 or type-2 herpes. It may or may not shorten an acute attack, does nothing against recurrences, and may possibly convert the virus to a more dangerous form. When this treatment was first used, however, there was no way to predict its usefulness. As with many treatments for herpes, only time and good studies will tell. I am afraid the money was wasted.

Forty-six-year-old housewife: "Four years ago, I developed herpes type-2. My life has been misery ever since that first attack. My husband won't come near me. He looks at me as if I'm dirty and hasn't touched me since he found out about the herpes. I don't even know how I caught this disease. Please send any information you have. I feel so lonely and ignorant."

Author's comment: This unfortunate woman is badly in need of an understanding and sympathetic physician and both she and her husband could benefit from a herpes self-help group or psychotherapy. I doubt that he will go with her initially, but as she becomes more confident and knowledgeable she may bring him around to being a more supportive mate. It may particularly interest both of them to know that *he is as likely to have introduced herpes into the home as she,* particularly as she does not know the source of her infection. Either partner could have had silent herpes smoldering for years before marriage or he, in fact, may have picked up a silent infection during an extramarital sexual encounter in the past. Her husband could then be blaming her for the illness he originally contracted and then passed on.

Twenty-eight-year-old male financier: "I have a really active sex life, or at least I used to have an active sex life. Now every time I have intercourse, I break out in blisters within two days. I know this is genital herpes, but what can I do to stop the attacks every time I have sex? My life is hell and the woman who gave it to me wasn't even worth the time of day!"

Author's comment: Many people report having had sexual intercourse within ten days of the onset of active recurrent genital disease. This young man certainly has a well-established cause for reactivation. He might try reducing sexual activity somewhat if he is terribly bothered by the recurrent infection, but most importantly, until specific treatment is available, he should inform his sexual partners that he may have active herpes. He should also use the contraceptive gel, condom, or other mechanical guards suggested later in this book in an effort to prevent further spread of his illness. With time, his recurrence rate stands a good chance of lessening, thus allowing him to return closer to his normal active sex life.

Twenty-two-year-old grammar school teacher: "My husband and I are expecting our first baby next month. The problem is that I have had genital herpes in the past, although no known attacks in two years. Is it safe for me to have my baby the regular way or should I have a cesarean section? We are so frightened that something bad will happen to our baby."

Author's comment: This is an area where fairly clear guidelines have been established by the medical profession. The most critical action which this young woman should take is to work closely with her obstetrician in watching for recurrent herpes. If there is no evidence of active infection, as concluded by examinations and Pap smears up to the time of delivery, many doctors will elect to allow their patients to deliver through the birth canal. If primary or active recurrent infection is suspected, cesarean section is the safest route. This is discussed in some detail later, with many case examples given.

> Thirty-two-year-old saleswoman: "Last summer I had an attack of herpes 'down below.' It hurt so much and looked so awful that I went to my gynecologist immediately. He told me I had venereal disease and that it would go away for a while but probably come back again. I was given some painkiller and told to stop 'sleeping around.' As there was nothing more he could do, I was not to come back for this problem again. I was so angry I swore I would never see another doctor again, but news of your work on a new drug (acyclovir) has given me hope. . . ."

Author's comment: This is an example of the unfortunate encounter a number of patients have with their physicians. It has been such a problem in some cases that I have discussed doctor-patient relationships separately below. You do need a doctor and you must never abandon seeking help from the medical profession because of a few bad experiences. All this is rapidly changing now as doctors not only learn more about herpes but as we develop more and more useful methods of dealing with it. We have specific and nonspecific therapy and we have very important advice and management programs concerning your sexual partners, yourself, pregnancy, and newborn babies. You can only hurt yourself and those you love by giving up the search for professional help. I think you will be surprised at the recent enlightenment among doctors and their willingness to help.

If, despite the foregoing comment, your doctor is not enlightened or helpful, find another one. This may be done through the telephone Yellow Pages under "Physicians-Gynecologists," by calling a local university or other medical center, or by calling your state medical society and asking for the names of doctors who treat gynecologic (female) or urologic (male) problems.

> Fifty-six-year-old forklift operator: "When I was eight years old, I got herpes in my right eye and lost my vision. For the past year, I have had chronic herpes in my left eye

and now I am legally blind. I have lost my job. Please help me. I hear a corneal transplant can give me back my sight."

Author's comment: Patients with ocular herpes are among the ones whom we can help the most. We have specific treatment for each attack of infectious ulcers and we have cortisonelike drugs which occasionally must be used to decrease scarring. Unfortunately, despite all this, a very few patients go on to blindness due to clouding of the front of the eye as this man did. But he is correct in saying that a corneal transplant can give back his sight. Our success rate in restoring vision is now between 70 and 90 percent of all first operations. And if the first transplant fails for some reason, it can be repeated, with chances of success still being good. Such surgery, however, should be done only by an ophthalmologist skilled in transplantation work and particularly familiar with herpes.

Twenty-six-year-old female secretary: "My life has been ruined by this herpes. I am always depressed. I don't go out anymore because I am afraid to touch anyone. How can I tell anyone? I know I'll lose my job if my employer finds out. Sometimes I think about suicide. I can't help it. I feel so alone. Am I unclean?"

Author's comment: These letters and calls are the most worrisome of all and received all too often. This young woman is experiencing part of the "herpes syndrome" as discussed later. She has cut herself off from society because she feels guilty and unclean. Such withdrawal only distorts and unnecessarily worsens the early psychological effects of the illness. She very much needs to see someone trained in giving psychotherapeutic help and she needs to get herself out to join a herpes self-help group. It is essential that she realize that she is not alone, nor disgraced, and that there are many people who would like to have her join them in mutual support and companionship.

Thirty-eight-year-old computer repairman: "For years, I thought I could never have a friend or lover again. I avoided people because I had a venereal disease that couldn't be cured. My wife left me and took my kids. I thought it was all over for me until I read a newspaper article about HELP. I joined my local chapter (we have more than four hundred members) and my whole life changed. I have new friends. I understand about herpes. I am no longer afraid—and I can help others. . . . My girlfriend doesn't have herpes, but she comes to the HELP meetings. She understands my problem now too. Next month we are going to be married. . . ."

Author's comment: This, of course, is the most encouraging type of communication that we can receive. This man has successfully passed through all the early and unpleasant stages of the "herpes syndrome" and gone on to achieve a balanced normal life. He has done nothing that cannot also be done by every other person discussed above. The existence of many more support groups, physician awareness, and new treatments will serve to make their way easier. Over the years, I have seen a shift in the balance from the more morose and severely depressed patients to those actively seeking and obtaining help both on the social and medical fronts; the swing of the pendulum will continue for the better.

While recurrent herpetic infections in the genital area are never as severe as a full-blown first infection, they are frequently far more distressing because of their repeated, often unpredictable timing. As you have seen above, and possibly felt yourself, such recurring infections do cause tremendous feelings of anger, guilt, anxiety, and depression. Sex lives and marriages have been ruined because one mate treats the other as a pariah, an evil person to be avoided. Other patients withdraw socially, for fear of spreading their infection. This only increases the mental anguish of the sufferer. Much of this unhappiness could be avoided if patients and their partners would simply think logically about the nature of the disease. *There should be no shame or guilt associated with genital herpes.* People do not acquire it while committing crimes against society. They acquire it during the course of making love, a perfectly normal and reasonable human need. The tragedy of venereal herpes, then, is not that it is a disease spread because of sexual activity and love, but that the person who has it may suffer recurring discomfort and unsightly disease. Emotional support should be given to relieve any associated feelings of guilt; many people already have enough to contend with in the physical nature of their disease.

The Emotional Impact of Genital Herpes on You and Your Doctor: Why Things Go Wrong and How to Make Them Right

As we have seen, herpes simplex infections cause a wide variety of emotional reactions which include frustration, anger, guilt, helplessness, fright, and depression. You will experience these feelings most commonly and intensely if you have genital or eye disease, but they may also come at any time with other forms of herpes. If you have chronic genital sores or a scarred eye, it may seem trivial that a friend woke up with his or her mouth totally surrounded by a mass of red, raw blisters. But suppose your friend has to give the biggest public sales presentation of her lifetime that day and her career is riding on it—or perhaps your friend was planning to "pop the question" to his girlfriend that evening. Can you imagine that their reactions would be much different from yours at that moment in time?

The usual term we give to any of you in situations such as the above is "psychologic stress." You certainly do not need to have herpes to have this kind of stress. Six out of every ten Americans are under obvious psychological stress just from the trauma of normal, everyday life. If you add onto this burden the effects of having herpes, the stress factor rises immensely and your emotional reactions with it.

Suppose, then, that you go to see a doctor about some painful blisters. Your physician makes the correct diagnosis of herpes—and then what? It is not simply a matter of writing out a prescription and sending you on your way with the answer to your problems: a cure for herpes. Your doctor looks at you sitting there—unhappy, feeling sick, and desperately wanting both medical help and emotional support. What can be done? Unfortunately, family physicians already spend about one fifth of their time providing psychological support. But remember, for some this is not their area of expertise, either by training or experience in actual office practice. It is only natural, then, that a few physicians are uncertain of their own ability to manage the emotional aspects of your illness or are perhaps too busy treating "real sickness" to offer you much help with your feelings about the whole event.

If you happen to have been examined by a doctor who is not comfortable treating herpes, the following may have happened to you. The message of your doctor's feelings of helplessness and/or "disinterest" came across to you all too clearly. Immediately, new psychological difficulties arose which affected your relationship and interactions with your physician. You were not only upset and angered by your own illness, but you may have felt betrayed by your physician's apparent inability to help you, either medically or emotionally. You may even have felt that your doctor wanted nothing to do with you because you had done something "unclean" or that you were being punished for some wrongdoing in life, real or imagined. And thus begins a vicious cycle. Your strong emotions are fed right back to your doctor, consciously or unconsciously, and you may have induced in him the same terrible feelings you were sensing in yourself. Doctors are human too and, as we have noted, not always able to concern themselves with the psychological aspects of illness, particularly when their medical resources are limited. You may well have found that instead of sitting down with you and discussing the things that you can do to help yourself and those close to you in terms of mental and physical well-being, your doctor just informed you that "There is no treatment for it," or "You have to learn to live with it," and "Good-bye."

Such a discouraging attitude on a doctor's part is unfortunate, of course, but this is rapidly changing for the better as more specific treatment becomes available and as the medical community itself learns more about herpes. As you will read, however, there is a great deal that can be done even now. But you didn't know that when you first sought medical help. The effect of "learn to live with it" and "good-bye" may have served only to increase your despair and depression unnecessarily. If you allow yourself to become "hexed" by such a pronouncement, the predictions of a grim life may become self-fulfilling. Being sure that things will turn out badly is one of the best ways to assure that they will. As you will read under "Television and the Press: You Are Not Alone—The Personal Stories of Others," the personal stories of patients with genital herpes (or really any form of herpes) can be one of emergence from despair and isolation to a full life and rewarding relationships. Part of this growth will come from the support of friends, but, at least in the beginning, part must also come from your doctor.

The first thing that you should remember, then, is that while we can treat but can not cure herpes biologically at this time, there is much to be gained from the psychological support, sympathetic understanding, and practical advice that your physician can give, once a mutually satisfying relationship is established. Start with the assumption that your doctor may feel frustrated because he can not hand you a permanent cure. In addition, he feels the disappointment and despair that quite naturally comes from you. It may sound strange and as if "it shouldn't be this way," but *you* may have to be the one to set the doctor at ease initially, just to get the two of you off on a good working relationship. This will benefit you greatly in the long run.

As you and your doctor talk after the exam, don't be afraid to tell him or her of your own feelings of frustration and anger, but also let your doctor know that you understand that it is a tough problem, that you know there isn't any cure yet, and that you realize treating such illness can be as frustrating for the doctor as for the patient. But you have come to him or her for help and you need advice and support until a cure is found. A doctor who senses that you are willing to try and to listen, rather than to fight or ignore what advice he does give because it does not satisfy all your needs, is one who will be able to give you much help in all aspects of your illness.

What, then, can you expect from your physician in the way of help? He or she can be expected to:

1. explain the cause, physical appearance, and symptoms at various stages of the acute illness;
2. encourage open communication, particularly concerns you may have about the medical and social aspects of the infection;

3. give treatment to relieve the acute disease and the anxiety associated with it;

4. set up realistic treatment goals and make specific suggestions as to how you can attain them;

5. be prepared to assist you sympathetically and medically in achieving some control over recurrent disease;

6. inform you about and refer you, when appropriate, to promising new treatment breakthroughs;

7. involve, whenever possible, your family or close companions in understanding your illness and in encouraging you in dealing with it;

8. protect you from wasting time and money on useless unproven but sometimes financially exploited "cures" for herpes;

9. refer you, if it appears potentially useful, for such specialized techniques as insight psychotherapy and hypnosis and herpes support groups.

As your relationship to your family physician or psychotherapist (see "Regaining Your Self-Esteem and Social Life: Sources of Support and How They Work") grows stronger and more reassuring, you will find it easier to release the inner feelings which temporarily prevent you from achieving a wholesome sense of well-being. If your herpes is genital, you will vent and thus dissipate your anger and resentment against the sexual partner responsible for your illness. You will gradually be relieved of many of the terrifying feelings which strike at your most basic biologic and emotional drives, feelings which concern sex and love. You will no longer see yourself as physically and emotionally alienated from human companionship. You will be relieved of your sense of sexual isolation and lowered self-esteem. And as you become more comfortable with your illness and know what to expect, when to expect it, and what to do about it, your life will return to near normal and you will feel an inner peace that may have been missing for years.

As you grow stronger in your own abilities to cope with your herpes, you will need your doctor less and less for emotional support and more just for medical treatment when needed. You may find, in fact, that you could well serve as support and succor for another friend with herpes, a friend who is just starting to travel the long road down which you have just passed.

Television and the Press: You Are Not Alone—The Personal Stories of Others

During the past few years, herpes has attracted national attention on television, radio, and in newspapers and numerous magazine articles. The discovery of this new epidemic disease has, on rare occasion, been parlayed into sensationalized articles focusing on pain, physical disfigurement, damage to newborn babies, and the apparent helplessness of the medical community. These articles, while clearly the exception to the rule, have undoubtedly been a source of some anguish to those of you who have had the illness and a source of distinct discomfort to those of you who fear contracting it.

Fortunately, the news media in general have played a very responsible and important role in familiarizing a previously poorly informed public audience about this medical problem. Articles and programs focused on herpetic disease have emphasized not only the nature of the illness itself, how it is contracted, past and present attempts at therapy, and the assistance you may expect to receive from the medical community, but the fact that patients with genital herpes are not alone in their plight. Great attention has been paid to telling you, the public, the personal stories of many patients who have this illness. Sadly, not all of these stories are pleasant to hear, but they clearly convey the message that any suffering you may have as a result of this infection is shared by thousands of other people just like you and many of them have learned to cope with their illness in such a manner that they have returned to essentially normal lives. The public presentation of the personal lives of these people has made it clear that many patients with herpetic disease pass through the same period of anger, withdrawal, and depression before ultimately learning to cope with their illness. They serve as models to any of you who may be at earlier stages in coming to terms with your infection. In each of the articles discussed below, one or more points must ring true with any of you who have had herpes or those of you who worry about getting it. Some points of discussion are painful, but many offer hope through the media's excellent and balanced coverage of this epidemic illness.

On November 2, 1980, the Chicago *Sunday Tribune* had three major front headlines. One concerned the American hostages in Iran; the second, the Carter-Reagan election (just two days away); and the third, THE HERPES EPIDEMIC—INCURABLE "LOVE-BUG" DISEASE SWEEPS THE U.S. (Author: John Van). Inside was an article which accurately covered all major points concerning the illness, including herpes's two-thousand-year history, its present incidence of up to five hundred thousand new infections per year, the physical appearance of the infection, and precautions to be taken by pregnant women known to have the infection. There was some discussion relating the increase of sexual freedom to the appearance of the herpetic epidemic and a discussion of several new therapeutic approaches under investigation at that time. Of the six treatments discussed, only one, acyclovir, has since been FDA-approved. In an all too true statement, Mr. Van commented "because there is no proven cure for herpes, many patients go from physician to physician seeking relief, and many try home remedies."

Similarly, *People* magazine ran a bold headline A NEW AND IN-CURABLE VENEREAL DISEASE CALLED HERPES IS SWEEPING THE COUNTRY, and *Reader's Digest* warned about A GRIM NEW VENEREAL DISEASE IN OUR MIDST; both of these articles again documented many of the cold hard facts about genital herpes and again greatly assisted in public awareness but could not offer much hope of relief from the disease.

Time magazine on June 30, 1980, compared herpes to a disease feared by all from biblical times until treatment was found in the twentieth century. HERPES: THE NEW SEXUAL LEPROSY—"VIRUSES OF LOVE" INFECT MILLIONS WITH DISEASE AND DESPAIR cried the magazine headline. In it, we learned about a young woman who contracted genital herpes because her doctor misinformed her about the infectivity of the disease. We also read of a young man who was divorced after contracting herpes during a single sexual encounter while on a business trip. After passing the disease on to a new lover, he was quoted as saying, "I regard myself as a carrier of an invisible, incurable disease. I have a guilt trip that won't quit." A twenty-nine-year-old nurse and her new baby were separated on doctor's orders from other women in a maternity ward and isolated in a room marked ISOLATION: HERPES. She bitterly commented, "I felt so dirty, I had to figure out ways to keep the grandparents away from the hospital."

The same article reported that herpes had broken out of the lower classes and the "viruses of love" were now infecting entire college dormitories and riding "the waves of rising divorce and crumbling monogamy." While this article does not discuss what can be done to help the herpetic patient and those close to him or her, it does review the failure of several therapeutic approaches, thus warning the public against wasting time and money on useless medication. The article closes on a sad note familiar at that time to too many herpes patients. "After being told by a doctor that he had herpes, Ray, a reading instructor, turned on departure to shake hands; the doctor would not extend his."

While all of these stories ring true, it is clear that their effect on the reader should not be to instill a gross mistrust and anger against doctors, nor a fear that people with genital herpes are forever to be avoided. Their aim is to inform the public of the current state of this illness, to warn against useless therapeutic approaches, and to encourage patients in coping with their illness through exposure to those who have already mastered the many associated problems.

In a follow-up article published on August 2, 1982, *Time* reminded us again that "herpes, an incurable virus, threatens to undo the sexual revolution."

Recognizing the enormous and often unnecessarily painful emotional impact the illness could have, the authors explored to great extent the psychological phenomena experienced by many people with genital herpes and the various positive and negative attitudes adopted by them. Pertinent discussions by various physicians, researchers, and psychotherapists interested in genital herpes were interwoven among the personal stories. The closing statements of this article succinctly state the best possible approach to living with herpes: "Herpes is only as devastating as a patient allows it to be . . . Indeed, herpes is so dependent on mood and emotion that once a sufferer regains self-confidence, many outbreaks can be tamed and managed." We are as happy or as unhappy as we make up our minds to be.

Perhaps one of the most useful of the articles written on the psychology of herpes was Daniel Laskin's "The Herpes Syndrome," (New York *Times Magazine,* February 21, 1982. While Mr. Laskin most competently covered the current facts and figures on genital herpes, he also devoted a great portion of his article to the psychological impact of this illness in discussing what is now referred to as the "herpes syndrome." He described emotions which must be felt by all of you who have contracted this illness; that you may feel tainted, fear that no one will ever want to love you. You may be totally confused in terms of whether or how to tell new friends or prospective lovers about your infection.

Laskin takes us through the personal conflict, anguish and ultimate victory of a thirty-two-year-old architectural designer who contracted genital herpes. This young man suffered the classical "herpes syndrome." Initially, he felt "impaired, damaged." He withdrew from his friends and was ashamed. He went through a classic pattern of anguish and isolation for more than a year until he ultimately joined a herpes discussion group. This was the beginning of a major change for the better in this young man's life. He was quoted as saying, "When you can talk about a problem, you can begin to talk yourself out of it. The group made me feel less unique. It put things into perspective." Recurrences of herpes still complicated this man's social life, but he no longer felt compelled to cancel social arrangements because of a recurrence. Because he had learned to speak of his herpes, with those whom he trusted and who trusted him, he was never turned down by a prospective lover. He now looks on his illness as simply a "periodic annoyance, not an eternal curse." While his sex life has changed, we may feel that it is in some ways changed for the better. He is more selective about his sexual partners and places value more on emotional commitment and less on the quantity of sex. He predicts that the effects of herpes nationally will be to cause us to move toward fewer but deeper and better relationships.

Radio talk shows and television coverage have also provided excellent and, in many ways, a more personal contact with other people who have contracted genital herpes. "60 Minutes" ran a show clearly emphasizing the personal anguish and methods of coping which had been worked out by the several highly motivated guests from a genital herpes support group. They described fears shared by all patients who have this infection; fears of cancer, fear of infecting their babies, and fear of spreading the disease to other people.

On October 14, 1980, "Donahue", in a very fine program, invited guests from a local herpes support group, the national administrator of HELP, a division of American Social Health Association (ASHA), a lobbyist on venereal disease for the ASHA, and a physician who is an international expert on herpetic infection. Mr. Donahue introduced the problem by going straight to the heart of the matter for all people with this illness. "It's a tremendous physical problem, not to mention the emotional impact that herpes patients sustain. It alters sexual activity. It certainly must have an enormous impact on the person's self-worth . . . and much of the problem of herpes is made more complicated by the ignorance which surrounds it."

James (pseudonym), a genital herpes patient, told an all too familiar story—"And when I went to get some treatment, what happened was I was told a bunch of stories, and I went and researched the whole thing myself and found out there was nowhere to go, there is nobody going to tell me what was going to happen, and I thought, 'Oh my God, the whole biological part of my life is gone. What am I going to do?' And there was no one there for me to turn to."

When asked how he felt when he first found out the true nature of his problem, James responded, "Angry, frustrated. I really wasn't sure how to deal with the whole situation. So it took me, personally, about a year and a half to come to grips with the whole thing and say, 'OK. I can go out and do my thing.'"

When Mr. Donahue inquired concerning James's responsibility toward intimate contact, he replied, "You have to figure out how you're going to deal with this thing, so—not just for me, but from talking to the many people I've come in contact with. . . . If you have a date on the weekend, you are preparing on Monday. Friday, you're checking yourself out and, 'Oh, do I have a little pain in my left leg?' You want to make sure you are in really good shape. But at that point, you know, it's a few months after you get it."

Another guest on the show was a young woman, Sarah (pseudonym), who also told an all too familiar story of her first dealings with herpes. "I went to six doctors before the sixth one finally just looked at it and said, 'Yes. That's herpes.' . . . I spent two thousand dollars trying to find a cure for herpes with all these doctors and taking every possible medication for it. In the beginning, I was so angry that I wanted to take that money and just hire someone to put this guy [the source of her infection] away. I was very angry. And then I didn't know anything about it, so I didn't know if it was going to come back or if that was it. And it didn't come back until six months, and then it came back in that one spot. And then I had it six times. I've had it for three years and I had it six times the first year and six times the second year."

Sarah was then asked about how she handled her intimate relationships. "My relationships have changed, because I've really put a close watch on how I deal with people. I was always careful in the past, but I developed a friendship and a relationship first, and the quality of my relationship with people has become better, I think."

Sarah had finally sought help and counseling through the New York chapter of HELP. She gave an interesting description of her first meeting. "When people came to our first meeting, they wore dark glasses. I mean, people had no idea who they were going to meet at the meetings; they stayed in the back and it took a long time before they came forward. And most of our members are all like us."

Mr. Donahue commented on how reassuring it must have been to know that she wasn't alone.

"Absolutely. Of course, at first I was afraid and then I said, 'This is a big part of my life. This is who I am. I'm not Herpes; I'm Sarah and I have herpes.' And you really have to just understand what it is, you know, except it is just being part of yourself. It's nothing bad, there's nothing wrong with it."

Much of the remainder of this program was given over to discussions with Dr. Lawrence Corey as to the difference between type-1 and type-2 herpes, current therapy, the fact that there are between three and eight million episodes of genital herpes per year in the United States, and what can be done both to relieve the acute illness and to prevent its spread to sexual partners. An administrator and a lobbyist from the American Social Health Association gave practical information concerning support groups and what is being done in Washington to help patients with this illness. Telephone calls poured in from married couples, people trying new and unproved remedies, women concerned about their unborn children, and people just wanting to talk to others who had suffered the same problems with which they were coping.

The media has been, then, and will continue to be a very important source of information on herpetic illness. The coverage has largely been responsible and compassionate as well as accurate and with time we may hope that the headlines may one day read THE CURE FOR HERPES HAS BEEN FOUND.

Regaining Your Self-Esteem and Social Life: Sources of Support and How They Work

As we have become more aware of the extent of the herpes epidemic and the emotional toll it has been taking on those directly or indirectly involved, many people have turned to a variety of methods for re-establishing their self-esteem and coping successfully with an unexpected change in their lives. These methods include: 1) support groups; 2) individual talking psychotherapy; 3) group psychotherapy; 4) hypnosis and relaxation techniques; and 5) social introductory services and personal advertising.

1) *Support groups* have been mentioned in other areas of this book. Their importance in calling attention to the herpes epidemic and in offering assistance to those caught up in it can not be overestimated. The largest of these groups is the American Social Health Association (ASHA), which sponsors the HELP organization (Herpetics Engaged in Living Productively). The vast majority of HELP members and administrators are themselves people with genital herpes. In addition, there are local HELP advisory groups which are made up of physicians and psychotherapists specializing in the diagnosis and therapy of herpes of all types.

In highly populated states such as California and New York,

the membership numbers in the hundreds if not thousands, with many large chapters. In smaller states such as Massachusetts, an initial group was put together composed of members from most of the New England states, with the meeting area being Boston. Once the group was set up and the size of the membership recognized, smaller groups split off from the main Boston organization to form their own chapters within their separate New England states. This has been true throughout the country with larger HELP organizations often serving as the source of a nuclear group which, once established, then grows in membership in more rural areas. Some of the major cities and states where there are chapters are listed below; there are many other smaller subdivisions in other cities and states which may be located by contacting the central office in Palo Alto, California. As some of the chapters may change locations, the Palo Alto headquarters should be contacted for the most recent addresses.

HELP LOCAL CHAPTERS*

ALABAMA
  Montgomery
  Birmingham
ARIZONA
  Phoenix
CALIFORNIA
  Herpes Resource Center
  American Social Health
    Association
  National Headquarters
  P.O. Box 100
  Palo Alto, CA 94302
  Inland Empire (Los
    Angeles suburbs)
  Long Beach
  Culver City

  Orange County—Yorba
    Linda
  Sacramento
  San Diego
  San Francisco
  San Francisco/East Bay
  San Francisco/South Bay
  Santa Barbara
  Whittier
COLORADO
  Colorado Springs
  Denver/Boulder
CONNECTICUT
  Greater Hartford/New
    Britain

* Reproduced, in part, from *The Helper* vol. 4, no. 2, June 1982 (quarterly publication of the Herpes Resource Center).

DISTRICT OF
  COLUMBIA
  Washington
FLORIDA
  Palm Beach
GEORGIA
  Atlanta
HAWAII
  Honolulu
IDAHO
  Boise
ILLINOIS
  Chicago
KANSAS
  Kansas City, Missouri
LOUISIANA
  New Orleans
MARYLAND
  Baltimore
MASSACHUSETTS
  Boston
MICHIGAN
  Tri-City
    (Saginaw/Midland/Bay
    City)
  Detroit
  Flint
  Grand Rapids
  Lansing
MINNESOTA
  Twin Cities
    (Minneapolis/St. Paul)

MISSOURI
  St. Louis
  Kansas City
NEW YORK
  Buffalo
  Long Island/Port Jefferson
  New York City
NORTH CAROLINA
  Triangle
    (Raleigh/Durham/
    Chapel Hill)
OHIO
  Cincinnati
  Cleveland
  Columbus
  Toledo
OREGON
  Portland
PENNSYLVANIA
  Philadelphia
  Pittsburgh
TEXAS
  Dallas
  Houston
WASHINGTON
  Olympia
  Seattle
  Tacoma
WISCONSIN
  Milwaukee

The purpose of the HELP organization is not one of formal psychotherapy. It serves rather as a source of the latest information on herpes, the organizer of group meetings for the dissemination of this information, and a setting within which you can meet other people who have been or are involved with someone with genital herpes. Such social contact in itself provides much relief from isolation and serves for the exchange not only of medical information but information as to what problems other people have had with herpes and how they have handled them.

Two additional and very important services are provided by HELP. One is the publication from the Herpes Resource Center of a quarterly newsletter, *The Helper,* which is sent out to all members and to local HELP advisory groups. This letter brings members up to date on recent developments in herpes research, as well as in the diagnosis and treatment of various herpes-related conditions. The second additional service is the support of a Washington lobbyist who calls the attention of the legislators to the herpes public health problem. This, in turn, aids in the federal funding of medical and social research into herpes.

Perhaps the most difficult aspect of joining a HELP organization is similar to that encountered in joining any group for the purpose of discussing such a personal problem as genital herpes —fear of being "found out." A number of HELP members have described the tremendous personal resistance which they had to overcome to make themselves go to a first meeting. They often wore dark glasses, despite the fact that the meetings were held at night, and stayed quiet and close to the back of the room in order to maintain the position of observer and not be noticed. As the informality and relaxed atmosphere of the meetings became apparent, however, they, in turn, relaxed. Over the course of time, they actively joined the group in discussion and herpes-related projects.

The meetings are run by members themselves, not by professionals, and there is no pretense that they are being held for therapeutic purposes, although this is an obvious beneficial byproduct from such social contact. Occasionally, formal meetings with professionals are arranged and announced, with a speaker invited to discuss some aspect of herpetic illness and its management. Perhaps the most important thing to remember in attending one of these meetings is that there is no one there who is not also infected with herpes or closely involved and sympathetic toward someone who has the illness. You will not be singled out, ridiculed, rejected or have your job put in jeopardy. You will, rather, find a receptive group with problems similar to your own and members at various stages in the process of learning to live successfully with herpes.

It is not uncommon for HELP members who have been extremely active in the organization eventually to master their illness so well that they ultimately leave the organization and return to their previous life-style. This may take one or two years but is an obvious goal and signifies a favorable turning point in the lives of many people with herpes infections.

The ASHA-HELP organization is not the only nonprofessional group formed for the purpose of mutual support among genital herpes patients. Many groups are being formed in cities and towns throughout the country. These groups are often known to your gynecologist or medical doctor, as well as to psychotherapists who have a special interest in herpes. A few inquiries and telephone calls may well turn up a group in your own location if there is not a HELP organization nearby.

2) *Psychotherapy,* like any other work area, has its own language and beliefs. It is often difficult for anyone not familiar with that common language or belief system to understand or to accept it as something potentially useful to them. First and foremost, you must understand that *you do not have to be mentally ill to benefit tremendously from seeing a specialist in psychotherapy.* There is a widespread misconception that you must be "ill" in some way if you are unable to handle all of your problems, including illness, yourself. You would probably be amazed to know how many normal, mentally healthy, and highly productive people go into short- or medium-term therapy, just for the purpose of working out one or two of life's unexpected stresses. Herpes infection clearly falls into this category. Unfortunately, many of our values and expectations of ourselves include self-reliance, independence, and a kind of "rugged individualism" that means we should never need help from anyone. This is often in conflict with our other value systems, as we pride ourselves on helping others. It seems appropriate to help others but embarrassing or a sign of failure to focus on our own difficulties. Those opposing values may make it difficult for us to seek someone else's advice and opinion. It is harder yet when we feel so overburdened, helpless, guilty, or confused about the source of the problem: genital herpes. Occasionally, we don't even know the "right" questions to ask or fear

ridicule for asking "silly" questions. It seems that we expect to be rejected for fear of having done something wrong or not knowing the right answer. We assume that there is a "right" or "wrong" answer or life-style and we are the only ones who don't know it. Remember, nothing to do with emotional health and happiness is "carved in stone." We live in a world of gray zones, not black or white, and must work out which zones are best for our own gratification and healthy functioning.

The primary objective of psychotherapy is a change in the way you experience and handle on an emotional level your immediate problem: herpes. This results in an increasing ability to live more fully, both in the present and in planning for the future. This is done most commonly by "talking therapy." Such therapy may be given by psychiatrists, clinical social workers, or clinical psychologists. The differences among these three professions are not always clear in people's minds. There are, in fact, simple ways to find out about therapists. Training degrees, for instance, tell you to which profession a therapist belongs. A psychiatrist has an M.D. and has been educated as a physician. He or she has been trained in medical school in the practice of medicine and surgery. Specialized training in understanding and managing psychiatric illness comes after medical school. Unlike psychologists and social workers, psychiatrists may prescribe psychiatric medications. If you elect to see a psychiatrist, you should ascertain that he or she is "board certified" or at least "board eligible." This means that proper training in a recognized psychiatric institution has been successfully completed.

Clinical social workers usually have masters degrees (M.S.W.), although some also have doctorate degrees (D.S.W.) or degrees as doctors of philosophy (Ph.D.). Instead of medical school, these psychotherapists have their graduate education in schools of social work. Clinical, or psychiatric, social workers are trained in techniques similar to those used by psychiatrists. They are fully qualified, therefore, as therapists both for individual treatment and for group work. Not being physicians, however, they do not prescribe medication or make medical judgments. In selecting a clinical social worker as a therapist, you should ascertain that he or she is a member of the Academy of Certified Social Workers (ACSW). This indicates certification by a national professional group after four years of clinical training and experience following the successful completion of a national written examination. In addition, some states have now started requiring that social workers be licensed. This is additional indication that the person with whom you are entering therapy is a qualified psychotherapist.

Psychologists are trained at postgraduate institutes of psychology and receive master's and/or Ph.D. degrees. As a rule, a master's degree in psychology does not qualify that person to perform clinical psychotherapy. Even a Ph.D. in psychology does not indicate that the psychologist has necessarily been trained as a clinician. Many psychologists do have extensive clinical training and experience in patient management and therapy, but others are trained almost exclusively in research and may or may not have obtained clinical experience after the Ph.D. degree has been received. It is important to ascertain that the psychologist you consult is, in fact, a clinical psychologist with experience in talking psychotherapy.

The fees charged by psychotherapists are often of concern to many people. As a rule, psychiatrists, clinical social workers, and psychologists are covered by most medical insurance up to a certain dollar amount each year. Massachusetts Blue Cross-Blue Shield, for instance, allows $500 annually for psychotherapeutic services. In our society, we often erroneously think that quality means high costs. This is not necessarily true. Some therapists charge only high fees, while others are more flexible. Generally, clinical social workers have sliding fee scales, depending on your means and what they feel would be appropriate to your therapeutic needs. Psychiatrists and psychologists may or may not be flexible in altering their fee structures. It is important to establish the fee schedule early in your therapy so that there are no unpleasant surprises several weeks or months into your treatment. Ask about fees on the telephone during your inquiry or certainly during your first visit.

While the fee schedules are important, this should not be your only concern in selecting a therapist. It is very important that a suitable match be made between you and the person with whom you elect to work. It is a very good idea to obtain the names of two or three good therapists who are interested in helping people with herpes and have a consultation interview with two or more of them before making your final selection.

There are several ways to locate psychotherapists. One is simply to ask your medical doctor whom he or she thinks might help you in handling the emotional stress which accompanies herpes. Another source is to ask any friends who have been in treatment or who are themselves therapists. A third excellent source is the Yellow Pages telephone directory. The listings which you should investigate include: "Psychotherapists," "Psychologists," "Psychiatrists," "Social Service Agencies," and "Social Workers." You may also gain useful information by telephoning a local college, university health center, or community health center and request the names of qualified specialists in the field of mental health. In addition, many professional organizations maintain lists of qualified psychotherapists. Such organizations include state medical societies or psychology organizations, as well as local state listings of the National Association of Social Workers. The American Social Health Association also maintains referral lists, which are available through its local HELP chapters. The national address is given earlier in this section.

Because many people have had difficulties sorting out the maze of available therapies and choosing a person most compatible with them, both in terms of personalities and fees, psychotherapy referral centers have been formed in a few cities. These referral centers have lists of licensed psychiatrists, social workers, and psychologists, and usually specialize in arranging meetings between you and a psychotherapist who has a particular interest in your problem. In this instance, of course, it would be useful to mention your difficulties with herpetic illness. For a fixed fee, usually around $50, you will have a one-to-two-hour placement interview, as well as additional interviews with different recommended psychotherapists. You may then select the one who best meets your personal and financial needs.

In a recent article in the Boston *Globe* (June 24, 1982), Dorrit Gary related the experience of one young woman with such a service. The referral center had recommended a social worker because the fee schedule was most compatible with what she could pay. She had, however, a bias against social workers and requested that she see a psychiatrist first, then a psychologist, and finally the social worker. After comparing the three, she found that the social worker was, in fact, the "warmest and most sympathetic and I ended up liking her most." Another young man was also referred to three therapists for initial interviews. He felt that the first therapist was too young and made him uncomfortable. The second therapist was a psychiatrist whom he felt was "nonthreatening, perceptive, and a gentleman, about five years older than myself. He was involved but not overbearing. I chose him and didn't even go to see the third."

In making the decision to seek psychotherapeutic help for your feelings about herpes, it is important for you to know what to expect once in therapy. Recently, the mental health professions have shown much interest in time-limited forms of therapy and "crisis intervention." This therapy, which is often well-suited to problems such as herpes, is specifically oriented toward your illness and typically lasts from two months to one year. The average duration of treatment is four months. You usually meet with your therapist once weekly in face-to-face interviews. Your therapist will encourage rapid development of a good and productive working relationship between the two of you which will enhance your motivation and positive attitude. Such meetings will give you the support you need from someone who is sympathetic and understanding but who also has specialized knowledge and competence during a crisis period. The goal is the restoration of or increase in your sense of well-being by providing you acceptance and someone upon whom you can depend during a period of need as you deal with guilt, shame, depression, withdrawal, anxiety, or any other undesirable emotional reactions which may have entered your life. During the course of therapy, you will become more aware of yourself as "me" and discard the concept of yourself as an "herpetic." You should experience, to some degree, the caring and understanding of your therapist. Your perception of this will be based partly on your discussions but often through other less obvious cues, such as tone of voice and body posturing. As the relationship between you grows, you will deal more readily with what you are feeling immediately and the perceptions you have of yourself. As you come to experience fully the awareness of your feelings, you will be able to develop methods of coping with them. Your image of yourself will keep changing throughout therapy and reorganize to absorb and successfully handle previously highly stressful experiences and thoughts. As you pull your thoughts and feelings together and understand them, you will have less to defend and be able to process what is happening to you more accurately. This, in turn, will make you more effective in meeting and coping with the new problems brought on by herpetic illness and in handling personal and business relationships. Virtually all forms of tension, not just those related to herpes, are usually reduced, producing both mental and physical relaxation. Your behavior comes more under your own control as it matures in its understanding of your emotional reactions to illness and this will help you relate better both to yourself and to those around you.

3) *Group psychotherapy* is another form of treatment which you may elect to enter, rather than individual talking therapy. Many of the benefits are the same and often the choice simply comes down to whether you would rather meet individually with a therapist or with several other people who have a problem in common with you, namely herpes. This form of treatment involves the putting together of a group of people who have been emotionally stressed by the unexpected change in their personal health. The group is guided by a trained psychotherapist with the purpose being that each member of the group will help the others effect changes in their emotional reaction to the illness. Group sizes range from as few as three members to as many as fifteen. The best size, however, is usually between eight to ten people. Too few members results in too little interaction and too large a group may result in a confusion in the exchange of ideas and support. Group members are themselves the main source of cure and change for each other. The role of the therapist is to guide the group in productive functioning without controlling its interaction. Self-reliance is encouraged and the therapist will help you to gain in self-esteem and to function well as a member of the group. The therapist's role is also to keep discussions pertinent to the problem at hand—living with herpes—and to turn the discussion away from material which is not relevant or useful to that subject.

Each session, as a rule, lasts between one to two hours and the number of meetings may range from six to as many as thirty once-weekly meetings. With the exception of everyone having a common problem with herpes, the group may be quite mixed in the variety of members. This means people from all races, socioeconomic levels, ages, sex, and educational backgrounds. In some instances, however, small groups may elect to meet because they not only have herpes in common but because they have other factors in common such as sex, sexuality, social or educational common bonds. The advisability of which type of group is best for you will be largely determined by the group therapist during a preliminary interview.

The benefits to be realized by group membership are that you come to know that you are not alone in having a particular emotional problem or problems and that there are many ways of struggling with and coping with similar problems. In addition, you will feel a certain cohesion with your group members. You obtain a feeling of belonging after having been through a period of social isolation and possibly rejection. There is often a feeling of group loyalty and friendliness which develops as people come to work together and to move toward achieving a common goal: living successfully with a recurrent illness. There is often great security in such a cohesive group and this security provides relief from anxiety. In addition to security, however, membership in such a group inevitably results in certain group pressures which will move subtly in the already avowed group goal of a return to high self-esteem and an emotionally satisfying life. You will not be allowed to slip back into depression or withdrawal from your "team." You will receive continuous reinforcement, which includes group approval, that will motivate you to develop and maintain a new and better pattern of behavior.

Perhaps one of the most important uses of group therapy, at least at the beginning of your treatment, will be the opportunity for ventilation and release of inner tensions through the free expression of your innermost fears and secrets. Through this closed but public discussion with group members, such ventilation of feelings leads to relief of guilt and anxiety through talking. This, in many ways, relieves your own burden by sharing it with others, further enhances your association with your group members, and helps them in understanding you better through receiving information about your innermost thoughts and fears. All of this can be rapidly and effectively therapeutic.

4) *Hypnosis* has become an important adjunct to both individual and group talking therapy. The hypnotic state is an altered form of thinking which is not sleep but rather a heightened concentration on a specific problem or task with obliteration of all peripheral thoughts. The advantage of hypnosis is that it speeds up the impact of the psychotherapeutic process. The connection between skin disease and internal emotional conflicts is widely recognized but not well-understood. Hypnosis and relaxation training have been widely used for treating a variety of skin disorders. Most recently, this therapy has been turned toward treating patients with genital herpes. Not all patients have the capacity, however, for the intense concentration that can be structured and channeled by the hypnotist in efforts to accelerate psychotherapy. Like psychotherapy in general, hypnosis may be carried out on an individual basis or in groups. In selecting a hypnotist, you would follow the same channels suggested for the selection of a psychotherapist, but ask for someone with specialization in the use of hypnotic techniques as well as an interest in herpes.

In the work done using hypnosis in people with genital herpes, hypnosis has often been useful in relieving much of the symptomatology such as itching, pain, and burning. In addition, peripheral fears of passing the infection to a lover or newborn child and the fear of cancer may be brought under control and handled successfully. Although there is no conclusive data available, hypnotists working with herpetic patients report that the results are most encouraging and that people not only feel much better about their illness but frequently have experienced fewer and less severe recurrences of their herpes. You should be aware, however, that this is not true of every patient. Should you elect to use hypnosis in addition to psychotherapy as you seek to master your herpes, do not be discouraged if there is no actual change in the physical manifestations of the illness. Much of this is beyond your emotional control. What is not beyond your control, however, is how you feel about the illness. An apparent inability to reduce the frequency or severity of recurrences should not lead to feelings of failure. Hypnosis may be highly useful in re-establishing your emotional well-being, but it is not a physical cure.

5) *Introductory services and personal advertising* for people with genital herpes are perhaps the most recent addition to the methods of re-establishing a good social life.

The concept of a formal social introduction service, per se, is well-established in this country. Many of these services are computerized and do an excellent job of pairing people with common interests and backgrounds—or different ones, if that is what is desired. Advertisements for subscribing to these services are commonly run in daily and weekly newspapers. Joining a service is merely a matter of calling or writing to the service described in an advertisement, filling out the personal information card which is sent to you, and receiving the names and addresses of other members of the service who best fill your needs as you have stated them. You then contact, or are contacted by, one or more of these people and make the desired social arrangements.

Herpes introductory services are no different from the usual ones already established, except that you have one more thing in common: herpes. Dating someone who already has the virus and who knows that you have it too immediately relieves any guilt or fears that you may have about giving it to someone who does not have it. Herpes becomes a relatively minor issue in such a relationship and establishing a satisfying social life is the goal to be obtained. In fact, some people who have met through such services have found their herpes infections to be a positive factor in establishing many common bonds together.

The services themselves are still relatively small because they are new, but printed pamphlets announcing their existence and how to join are already available. These pamphlets are sent to gynecologists, urologists, dermatologists, psychiatrists, clinical social workers, and clinical psychologists, as well as to hospital clinics and services concerned with infectious disease or any of the above specialties. This information is often made available in waiting rooms or, if not out on a table, may usually be obtained merely by asking your doctor or medical office assistant. These services may also be advertised in the daily and weekly newspapers or magazines in your locale. One herpes introductory service founded by a patient with genital herpes started with just a few names but rapidly grew to the hundreds. It is not yet computerized, but the matching is done by personal review by the

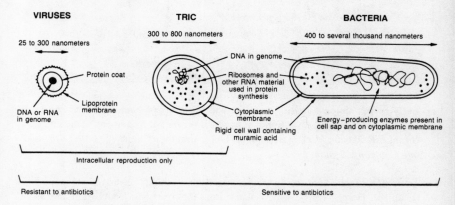

VIRUSES

25 to 300 nanometers

Protein coat

Lipoprotein membrane

DNA or RNA in genome

TRIC

300 to 800 nanometers

DNA in genome

Ribosomes and other RNA material used in protein synthesis

Cytoplasmic membrane

Rigid cell wall containing muramic acid

BACTERIA

400 to several thousand nanometers

Energy – producing enzymes present in cell sap and on cytoplasmic membrane

Intracellular reproduction only

Resistant to antibiotics

Sensitive to antibiotics

Key differences among various families of infectious organisms. Herpes organisms are in the viral family and cause the diseases discussed in this book. TRIC germs can cause eye infections and a venereal disease similar to gonorrhea, and bacteria can cause venereal (gonorrhea, syphilis) as well as a wide variety of nonvenereal infections. *(From P. R. Pavan, M.D., International Ophthalmology Clinics 15, Little, Brown and Company, Boston, 1975.)*

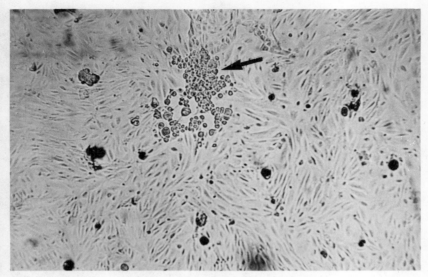

ABOVE

Early herpes simplex causing swelling and blistering of human cells grown in tissue culture (arrow). An antiviral drug would prevent further spread of the virus. *(From P. R. Pavan, M.D.*, International Ophthalmology Clinics *15, Little, Brown and Company, Boston, 1975.)*

BELOW

Twenty-four hours later the layer of cells is almost entirely destroyed for lack of treatment. Herpes virus can be isolated from the overlying feeder fluid and its type, 1 or 2, determined. *(From P. R. Pavan, M.D.*, International Ophthalmology Clinics *15, Little, Brown and Company, Boston, 1975.)*

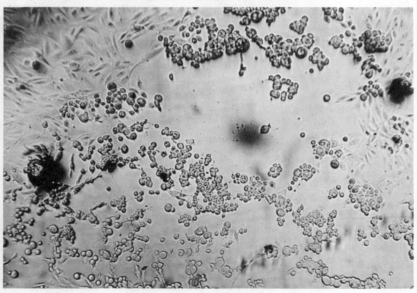

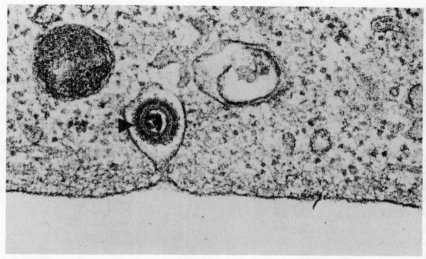

ABOVE

Infectious herpes simplex virus (arrow) invading a living cell wall. Note the three layers: an outer membrane, middle protein layer, and a dense central DNA genetic core. All herpes viruses — simplex, zoster, CMV, and E-B — look alike. (*Courtesy A. B. Nesburn, M.D., Journal of Virology 3, 1969.*)

BELOW

Life cycle of a typical herpes simplex virus during the active reproductive stage. In latency the viral DNA would just reside quietly in the nucleus without activating cell manufacture of new viral parts, as in step C above.

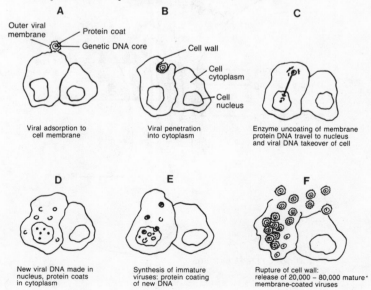

A
Outer viral membrane
Protein coat
Genetic DNA core

Viral adsorption to
cell membrane

B
Cell wall
Cell cytoplasm
Cell nucleus

Viral penetration
into cytoplasm

C

Enzyme uncoating of membrane
protein DNA travel to nucleus
and viral DNA takeover of cell

D

New viral DNA made in
nucleus, protein coats
in cytoplasm

E

Synthesis of immature
viruses: protein coating
of new DNA

F

Rupture of cell wall:
release of 20,000 – 80,000 mature·
membrane-coated viruses

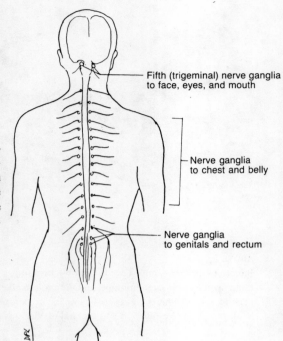

Location of sleeping herpes viruses in nerve ganglia along spinal cord. When viruses awaken from latency, they travel the nerves to the skin, where the nerves end and the blistering disease results.

Fifth (trigeminal) nerve ganglia to face, eyes, and mouth

Nerve ganglia to chest and belly

Nerve ganglia to genitals and rectum

BELOW
Most common areas of herpes blistering on external female genitals (vulva).

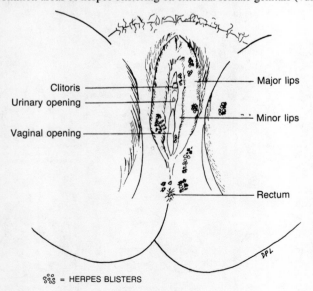

Clitoris

Urinary opening

Vaginal opening

Major lips

Minor lips

Rectum

= HERPES BLISTERS

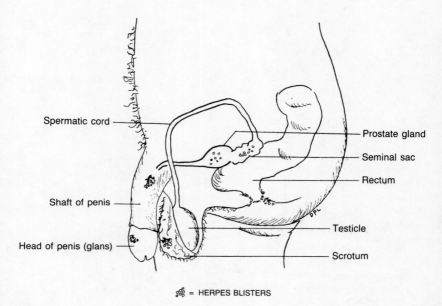

Spermatic cord

Prostate gland

Seminal sac

Rectum

Shaft of penis

Head of penis (glans)

Testicle

Scrotum

℄ = HERPES BLISTERS

ABOVE
Most common locations of herpes virus in internal and external male genital system.

BELOW
Female internal genital system showing silent herpes blisters on cervix.

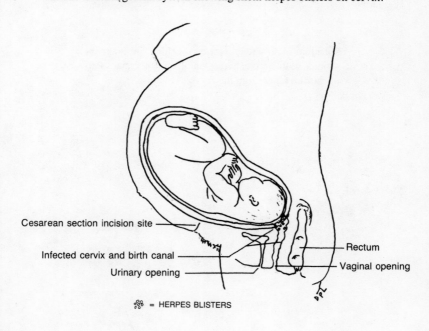

Cesarean section incision site

Infected cervix and birth canal

Urinary opening

Rectum

Vaginal opening

℄ = HERPES BLISTERS

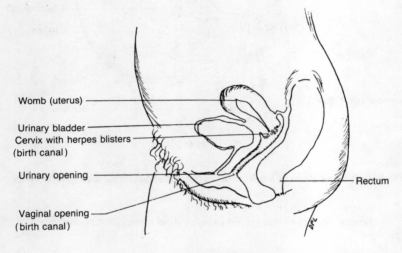

Womb (uterus)
Urinary bladder
Cervix with herpes blisters
(birth canal)
Urinary opening
Vaginal opening
(birth canal)
Rectum

°°° = HERPES BLISTERS

Location of cesarean section opening in pregnant woman with active herpes in the birth canal. Pap smears are taken from the cervix.

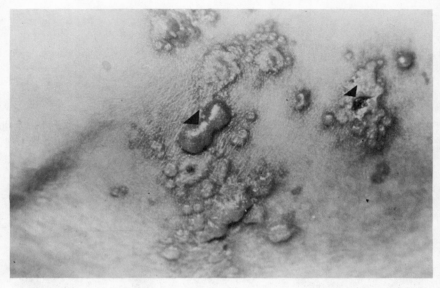

ABOVE
Herpes virus blisters in various stages of development. The large arrow points to a fresh, infectious blister. The smaller arrow shows early scab formation of the healing process. *(Courtesy Richard Whitley, M.D.)*

BELOW
Herpes simplex infection of the finger showing both blisters and scab formation. These sores may also occur in the nailbed.

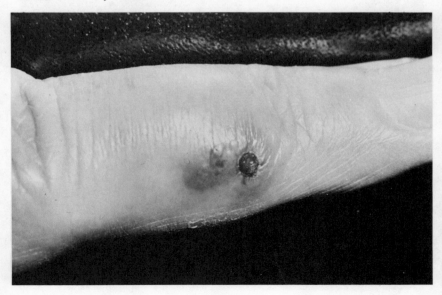

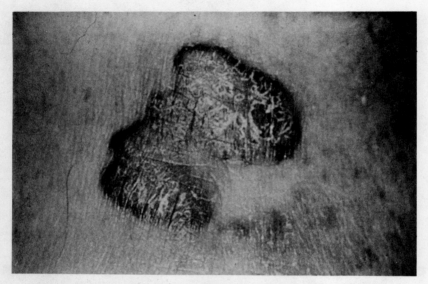

Kaposi's malignant sarcoma of the skin in homosexual patient with severe CMV (cytomegalovirus) infection. *(Courtesy Howard Baden, M.D.)*

founder and contacts made by giving members the names of those people who seem most compatible in terms of background factors other than herpes. At the rate many of these services are growing, some will soon be nationwide and provide a much needed solution to the self-imposed celibacy that many people with genital herpes have placed upon themselves.

Advertising is another useful means of contacting other people with genital herpes. These are usually listed in the "Personal" columns of weekly newspapers or local magazines. One such notice run recently was "HERPES-2. Two professional men—single, thirties—wish to meet women with same concern and an interest in theater, dining, and sports. Contact Box _____" (newspaper mailing address given). Personal advertising, like introductory services, is a well-established concept in this country. The addition of herpes-2 is just one more common binding factor between two people. Using your herpes as a positive factor in re-establishing your social life can be a great turning point in successfully managing what could otherwise be a negative and unnecessarily isolating determinant in your life.

Informing Sexual Partners of Your Infection

If you are a known carrier of *genital* herpes type-1 or -2 (in other words, if you have been diagnosed as having the infection even once), you will do your sexual partner(s) a great favor by telling them of the possibility of infection. In fact, if you think back to how you felt when you just learned that you had herpes and no one had warned you and taught you about the precautions you should take, you might see telling prospective partners as a moral obligation.

As you learned in the section on "Television and the Press: You Are Not Alone—The Personal Stories of Others," most people are terrified of telling anyone that they have an herpetic genital infection. This is a totally normal response; no one wants to risk the chance of rejection, especially when it concerns love and sexual desire. Nonetheless, those people who ultimately came to cope best with their herpes were those who faced up to it and took a responsible position concerning their illness, both in attitude and in their physical actions. The net result was that their relationships with people were less superficial, more trusting and rewarding, and little compromise had to be made in the quality of love relationships in the long run.

Step one, then, is to form a good relationship with someone worth caring for. Once the relationship is there and you are emotionally comfortable with each other, you can broach the subject gently and casually by mentioning that some time ago you came down with a virus infection which occasionally returns on you. In general, you know when these recurrences will come (if you do) and that during those few days it is best for you not to be physically intimate or close with anyone. You may then go on to explain, if the moment is right, what measures you can both take to protect against an inadvertent spread of virus during a period when no evidence of active infection is present. Taken slowly, easily, and with confidence, anyone truly worth your caring for will not reject you. When you take the time to show that you care and are responsible, they should respond in kind.

They may then take precautions, such as those discussed below, when you are having sexual foreplay or intercourse. It would also be advisable for them to get a good physical examination (gynecologic for women, urologic for men), including blood tests for herpes antibodies to find out if they are already infected. This is particularly important for any woman who may ever become pregnant, as the method for delivery for the well-being of the baby may be affected.

What about telling people that you have oral herpes, type-1, around your mouth or face? Frankly, it does not carry the same potential emotional impact experienced with genital infection. In fact, oral herpes is so common that, no matter whom you informed about your oral infection, they would probably just say, "Oh, I have it too." Nonetheless, there is something that all people entering an intimate relationship should consider and act upon when appropriate. Cold sores on the mouth may usually be caused by herpes type-1, but this virus, as you have read, can be spread to the genital region during oral-genital sexual activity and cause an infection similar to that of type-2. Therefore, if your cold sores happen to be active or if your partner has signs of activity, even a little warning tingle, either put off your lovemaking for a few days or at least avoid oral contact of any kind if you cannot wait until the sores have healed. Even though type-1 infection of the genital region appears to have much less tendency to recur than does type-2, it is still an infection that we would all like to avoid if possible.

"Herpes Phobia" (Fear) and "Delusional Herpes"

Both "herpes phobia" and "delusional herpes" have been reported in the news recently. These reports need clarification, as the two conditions are confused by some people as one and the same problem.

"Herpes phobia" is a phenomenon quite different from delusional herpes. The latter occurs in people who want to use herpes as an emotional shield to handle other problems. A phobia or being phobic means that you are terrified by something very real but which normally would cause moderate to little concern.

There are two forms of "herpes phobia." The first is seen in people who actually do have genital or other forms of herpes but who channel all of their emotional energy into focusing on that one problem, blowing it up out of all proportion. These people with herpes have redefined their other unrecognized emotional concerns into a clearly recognizable one: herpes. They seek psychotherapeutic and medical help for their herpes but tend to defeat the benefit of any aid, as they want to continue to deal with a known infection rather than an unknown emotional concern.

The second form of "herpes phobia" occurs in people who are consciously and genuinely afraid of herpes. This includes those who have it and those who do not. It is not a true phobia in the psychologic sense but rather an exaggerated fear of a real illness.

Knowledge about the illness and how it can be managed or avoided successfully reduces the anxiety and fear. Again, unduly exaggerated fears on anyone's part may reflect emotional troubles in other areas and may be helped by professional psychotherapeutic intervention. These problem areas can be as simple as associating herpes with an earlier illness in a loved one who was disabled in ways that now worry the person with "herpes phobia."

"Delusional herpes" occurs in a very different group of people than those with herpes phobia. A well-known psychological phenomenon is manifested when a widely publicized happy event occurs and many people enjoy a positive association with it. There are some people in our population, however, who for various reasons are unhappy and have a need to associate only with negative events be they natural disasters or human tragedy. Some of these people are lonely and need to "belong" to a group, and others substitute an imaginary problem in order to avoid facing a real one they already have. Confessing to a crime they have not committed is one method of satisfying these needs and wanting to suffer from an infamous illness such as genital herpes is another. These people have a psychological condition which is known as "delusional herpes." They truly believe they have genital herpes when, in fact, they do not. These people may have very little or very extensive intellectual knowledge of what herpes attacks are like. Some have never had a physical examination during the period when they are allegedly having one of their recurrences. They see their doctors "in between attacks" and accurately describe what sounds like a herpes episode. Other people with "delusional herpes" do not avoid physical examination at times when they feel they are having a recurrence but simply do not believe the negative results or are convinced that the doctor is in error. A blood test will frequently reveal that these people have little to no antibody against herpes type-2 and sometimes none against type-1.

It has been explained that people with "delusional herpes" use their imaginary genital infection as an emotional shield. Because they "have this illness," they can not or do not carry out certain social functions. They use the illness as a shield behind which they may protect themselves from partaking in activities that they really would like to avoid or, in some cases, would like to join but have not been invited to do so. People with this problem probably do not suffer the same unhappy emotional experiences of those who truly have the infection, but they are certainly in need of and would benefit from professional counseling by a social worker, psychologist or psychiatrist. It is only when the real roots of the emotional problem have been uncovered that such a person may begin to face the fact that he or she does not truly have a herpes infection but is simply using it as a protection against something else; something which they will then learn to handle successfully in talking therapy.

6. THERAPY AND PREVENTION OF GENITAL HERPES

For the vast majority of people, treatment of genital and rectal herpes is still symptomatic. Treatment of the latter was discussed in the section on "Rectal Infection." In this section, however, recommendations for treatment will be discussed, along with a brief review of the pros and cons of the more widely publicized recent therapeutic approaches.

Minimizing Stress and Fever

One very good way to start helping yourself in coping with genital herpes is to determine what factors in everyday life seem to bring on attacks and then try to avoid or minimize those factors. Fever has already been mentioned as less important in reactivating type-2 virus than type-1. Nonetheless, as with type-1 disease, taking two aspirin or aspirinlike pills every four hours to prevent fever during illness may be an important preventive step. Such minor trauma to the genitalia as wearing tight underclothing has been shown to cause reactivation of disease. Switching to looser undergarments may actually stop recurrences. Emotional stress, whether premenstrual, work, or socially related, may be allayed by taking a minor tranquilizer during that stressful period if your doctor feels it would help. Sexual intercourse itself, of course, may cause reactivation. The answer is not to stop having intercourse, as such sexual isolation may induce reactivation itself. The answer is to maintain as normal a sex life as possible, taking precautions for a partner when necessary, and then to start general therapeutic measures at the first tingle suggesting recurrent infection. *Do not, however, have sexual relations when you or your partner is actively infected, even if the recurrence is only at the early tingling stage, and do not be afraid to inspect your own and your partner's genitalia for sores, just as a precaution.*

General Therapeutic Measures

The general therapeutic measures one may use, both to minimize the severity of disease and possibly to shorten its course on
occasion, include good hygiene, local anesthetics (numbing ointments), and drying agents. You should bathe the outside genital
area twice daily with mild soap and water and then carefully rinse
clean and pat dry. Facecloths and towels used for this should be
cleaned in hot water and detergent and should be used only by
you.

Your external genital blisters or ulcers may be made less painful and, some physicians feel, will dry more quickly by using saltwater sitz baths. This is simply soaking the genitals and rectum by
sitting in a basin of warm salt water, made with one tablespoon
table salt per quart of warm water, for five to ten minutes once or
twice daily. The small basin may be set on the floor or on a
sturdy hard chair. Bathing the external genitalia with soap may be
done at the same time as the sitz bath or separately in shower or
tub. Be sure to dry carefully after bathing or, as noted below,
your condition may worsen. If you have severe pain, your doctor
may prescribe numbing anesthetic (lidocaine) ointment during
the worst part of the disease.

But while there are many infections and conditions involving
the genital area for which soaking or sitz baths are often recommended, herpes infections of the genitalia may on occasion be
made worse by such treatment. Many patients with herpes are
tempted to try home remedies and may use such therapy. The following cases are included to inform you about the possible conse-
quences not only of *oversoaking* your herpetic lesions, whether
they are genital or oral, but also of spending the better part of
your day at the beach in a wet bathing suit.[8]

Two young women who experienced recurrences of genital
herpes infections monthly for one to two years' duration
were seen in an outpatient clinic because of an unusually severe attack of their disease. Both women had many ulcers involving the external genitalia and the area between the
genitalia and rectum. Further questioning revealed that each

woman had been swimming on a hot summer day and their bathing suits had been wet for the better part of that day. Within twenty-four hours, each patient noted the presence of multiple lesions to a much greater extent than either had experienced with previous recurrences.

Two other young women were admitted to a hospital, with a diagnosis of primary genital herpes infection. Each woman had noted a few painful lesions on one side of her external genitalia. Their gynecologists had recommended frequent warm sitz baths three to four times daily, each of twenty minutes' duration. Within two to three days of beginning such treatment, there had been marked spread of these painful sores. Examination revealed many inflamed ulcers with a bad smelling exudate and extreme tenderness covering the entire external genital area. The genitalia were greatly swollen and the cultures taken from the area grew out herpes simplex type-2. Treatment was based on keeping the infected area dry by frequent use of a light bulb under a blanket [this should *only* be done under the careful *supervision* of the *paramedical staff*]. Medication for pain was given for three days. Within one to two days, the pain, exudation, and swelling were greatly relieved and both patients walked comfortably out of the hospital three days after admission.

Two women with somewhat different problems gave a history of mild recurrent herpes of their mouths for more than ten years. For the itching of their blisters, they had each used hot, wet towel compresses, four to five times daily, thirty minutes each time. The blisters spread rapidly as they continued their home remedy. Herpes type-1 was cultured from the sores, the compresses stopped by the physicians, and the blisters healed within a week without other therapy.

As any of us who enjoys a nice long soak in the hot tub knows, such a luxury causes roughening of normal skin. If herpes virus is present in addition, new blisters may develop on the roughened area and local spread of the disease may occur. Because of this risk, wet compresses or sitz baths should be minimized, by any of you who have active herpes infection, to that duration and frequency just necessary for good hygiene, and the area otherwise kept dry unless your doctor is using a medicated ointment. Wet bathing suits should be changed for dry clothing as soon as possible, whether genital herpes is known to be active or not.

Drying agents include 5 percent salt ointment (table salt) or 4 percent boric acid ointment applied to the sores four times daily for five days. These ointments are available at drugstores and may assist somewhat in the healing or comfort.

It should be remembered, however, that the safest and best treatment of all for recurrent genital herpes is good hygiene—washing with warm soapy water, clean rinsing, careful patting dry, and *keeping the area clean and dry during the attack*. Specific drug treatment is discussed below.

Other local forms of therapy you may have heard of include the application of cotton balls soaked in alcohol, ether, or acetone. This too may cause the ulcers and blisters to dry up more quickly, but ether and acetone are *flammable, explosive, dangerous to breathe, and not safe for use unsupervised by a doctor*. Alcohol may cause further irritation of your skin for a while. This technique can be used for disease on the outside surfaces only and should never be applied internally. Such use of drying agents will not, of course, prevent another attack later but have been reported by some doctors as of some use in shortening the duration of the blisters and discomfort. Only your doctor should decide upon such treatment.

Antiviral Drugs and Other Forms of Treatment

Antiviral drugs* are only now coming into their own as useful treatment for viral infections. Because there is such a widespread and often devastating onslaught of illness, it is fortunate that the herpes viruses differ from most other viruses in one key aspect. When a herpes virus invades your cells, it provides some of its own enzymes which are necessary for its own replication. This

* You may know these drugs by different names. TM (TM) indicates the commercial name, but all generic and abbreviations are included for your information.

means that herpes can not rely entirely on the enzymes that your own cells have to offer. These viral enzymes are different from your own. Such dependence on virus-created enzymes makes it possible to develop drugs which interfere, in part or completely, with those special virus enzymes and thus block the reproduction of new virus. Almost all of the most useful drugs used are in the antimetabolite family and as you will see, their effectivity and toxicity depends a large part on how specific their action within your infected cells is.

IDU (Herplex,™ Stoxil,™ Dendrid,™ idoxuridine) and TFT (Viroptic,™ trifluridine, F_3T) are two of the earliest antimetabolites used and were developed in the early 1960s. They are extremely useful in treating herpes infection of the eyes and are both FDA-approved for this purpose (see "Herpes and Our Eyes —Keratitis and Iritis"). Unfortunately, these two drugs are also activated by enzymes found in healthy human cells. This means that they are not selective in their actions and will exert toxic effects not only against cells with virus in them but to a lesser extent against normal cells. Because of this toxicity, they can not be used intravenously for serious or widespread herpes infections because the side effects on your body can be worse than the disease itself.

Ara-A (Vira-A,™ vidarabine, adenine arabinoside) is another highly effective antiviral drug which is FDA-approved for treating herpes infections in the eye (see "Herpes and Our Eyes—Keratitis and Iritis"). In addition, because it is not as toxic as IDU or TFT, it is also approved for use intravenously in cases of herpetic encephalitis (brain infection). This drug is not totally without toxic side effects, but this toxicity is far preferable to allowing the ravages of herpes encephalitis to go untreated.

Several successful cases have been reported using this drug intravenously for a variety of very rare but severe herpes virus infections.[2] Six patients were successfully treated with intravenous vidarabine for such herpes infections as chronic zoster (shingles) infection of the skin which had smoldered relentlessly for eight months, cytomegalovirus (CMV) pneumonia (see "The Gay Population and Herpetic Infections"), herpes simplex encephalitis, severe herpes zoster in a patient with advanced cancer (lymphoma), and widespread herpes simplex infection in a patient on high doses of cortisone. Within two to four days after the start of vidarabine therapy, all patients stopped developing new blisters and began to improve dramatically. There were minimal toxic side effects from the drug, all of which reversed when the drug was discontinued. This study demonstrated vidarabine's usefulness in potentially fatal cases which previously would have been considered hopeless. You will find several similar examples of the use of vidarabine in other sections of this book. As you will see in most cases, vidarabine was highly successful, but in a few, even this drug could not control certain forms of herpetic infection.

As I have mentioned, the herpes viruses must rely on providing some of their own enzymes during their reproductive cycle. The discovery of these enzymes has led to the development of *revolutionary new drugs which activate specifically with the virus enzymes without interfering with your normal cell enzymes*. The most well known of these drugs are Zovirax™ (acyclovir, ACV) and bromovinyldeoxyuridine (BVDU).

Acyclovir specifically inhibits a herpes enzyme called "thymidine kinase." This drug is highly effective against herpes simplex type-1 and type-2 and against chicken pox-herpes zoster virus. Unfortunately, it appears to have little effect on cytomegalovirus (CMV). Throughout this book, you will find specific case descriptions where acyclovir has been used in treatment of herpes simplex infections of the genitalia, skin, mouth, eye, brain, lungs, and in the newborn. It has also been used successfully in severe chicken pox and herpes zoster infection. Unfortunately, it has not been so successful in its application against CMV infections, as seen in cases discussed under "The Gay Population and Herpetic Infections."

The results of one of the largest studies on the effects of acyclovir ointment in genital herpes simplex infections are now available and reveal much interesting information concerning: 1) the period of time that patients with various forms of genital herpes are infectious; 2) those who will benefit from the use of acyclovir ointments; and 3) those who should not use it and why.[9] Patients applied either acyclovir ointment or a placebo (ointment with no drug) to all their external genital sores four times daily using a gloved finger.† It was never applied internally. Primary (first herpes ever) or first genital episodes of disease were treated for seven days and recurrent episodes for five days. Investigators found that people with primary infection of the genitalia had a wider area of ulceration and higher levels of virus than those who were having their first attack of genital herpes but who had had a previous infection with another type of herpes virus elsewhere in their bodies. This suggested that previous infection with herpes simplex confers some partial level of protection on patients who subsequently contract type-2 genital infections. It is obvious, however, that a prior herpes infection does not confer complete immunity to infection with another form of herpes virus.

The *period of shedding of infectious virus* in patients with primary genital infections was seven days in those receiving no treatment and only four days in those receiving acyclovir. If a patient had had prior infection with herpes simplex elsewhere in the body, the virus-shedding time was about four days in the untreated patients and only one day in those receiving acyclovir. Additionally, patients with primary genital infections had reduced severity of symptoms and a shorter time to crusting of the ulcers when acyclovir was used. Patients who had recurrent rather than primary or first genital infection shed virus for two days if they were in the untreated placebo group and only one day if acyclovir was used. This may indicate the very short period of time that people with recurring infections may actually pass the virus on. The sores last longer than does the virus.

There was no significant effect on the duration of symptoms in either the treated or untreated groups regardless of the patients' sex, but the sores healed sooner in treated men than in treated women. In fact, women with recurrent herpes showed no significant response at all to acyclovir treatment.

In follow-up studies to determine the rate of recurrent disease in these patients, it was found that nearly three quarters of both the treated and untreated patients had recurrences within two to three months. Therefore, treatment had no effect on preventing another attack later. It was also noted that despite the presence of

† Commercially marketed acyclovir is a 5 percent ointment usually applied with a finger cot or rubber glove (for protection of the hands and prevention of spread elsewhere in the body) six times daily for seven days.

acyclovir ointment on the genital region, new blisters were able to develop on the mucous membranes and skin in the presence of antiviral therapy.

The finding that men with recurrent herpes benefited from acyclovir treatment more than women seemed to be due to the fact that treatment was started earlier in male patients. Because of this, new studies are now under way to test the results of earlier administration of treatment. These studies involve giving the patient ointment to take home, where he or she is to begin therapy at the very first sign of tingling or other sensation which indicates that a recurrence is about to take place.

Nonetheless, we cannot ignore the results of the present study which indicate that while acyclovir ointment is effective in the treatment of primary and first genital herpes infections, it has little to no significant effect on recurrent genital disease. It has been suggested that topical acyclovir might reduce transmission of herpetic disease, but it should certainly not alter either the practices of abstaining from sexual intercourse while the ulcers appear active or the man wearing a condom if the situation is dubious.

One very strong argument for not using acyclovir in any situation where it has not absolutely been proven useful is that drug-resistant viruses can easily emerge.[30] We now know that herpes viruses lacking in the enzyme which acyclovir needs for activation occur naturally in some people. Indiscriminate use of acyclovir would select out these resistant forms and encourage their spread. These resistant viruses would not, of course, respond to treatment with acyclovir, even if the disease spread to a new patient was primary at the time of therapy.

Despite some of the negative results of the above study, we should still be quite encouraged by what has been achieved thus far. The early therapy studies are well under way. Chemically modified forms of acyclovir are now being tested and found effective. Acyclovir itself is being investigated for delivery in a new ointment base and, as mentioned below, this drug is being tested and has already been found to be effective as a pill.

Acyclovir has recently been approved by the Food and Drug Administration for marketing in ointment form as the first effective therapy, not only for primary genital herpes infections but for skin infections in patients whose bodies are unable to fight the spread of herpes virus. This inability to control the spread of herpes through the body is usually because of an underlying disease such as eczema, poor nutrition, cancer, or because certain drugs which suppress the body's white blood cell defense system are being used in therapy. Use of acyclovir in chronically debilitated patients will be virtually lifesaving in many cases by preventing uncontrolled spread of infection. The presently approved formulation is not expected to affect the rate or severity of recurrences. Because the drug is so specific in acting just on virus-infected cells while bypassing your normal cells which lack virus enzymes, there are no significant toxic side effects with its use.

Additional encouraging findings, many now in stages of advanced human study, show not only that the drug works well as an ointment for the eye, skin, or mucous membrane, but that it is effective intravenously for widespread, life-threatening herpes infection. Life-threatening herpes is very rare but can occur. The following case is put in to show you how successfully we can now treat these previously often fatal infections.[46]

A sixty-eight-year-old man with chronic leukemia was admitted to the hospital for fever, chest infection, and a herpes cold sore on his upper lip. Despite intensive treatment with several antibiotics, neither his fever, pneumonia, or herpes improved. He became steadily more ill on antibiotic treatment and the herpes ulcers spread from his mouth to his tongue and back of his throat. Chest X ray was suggestive of a viral pneumonia. Antibiotic treatment was therefore discontinued and he was placed on intravenous treatment with acyclovir for three days. Within forty-eight hours, his fever was gone and he was up and walking about within a week. Two weeks later, he left the hospital feeling well and all herpes ulcers were healed. There was no sign of any toxic side effect during the period when he was treated with the acyclovir.

Although the initial studies are just now being carried out, we have already learned that acyclovir may be given to normal people as a *pill* and that there will be excellent absorption of the medication from the intestinal tract, resulting in blood levels which would be effective against herpes infection. The following is one of the first clinical studies carried out using such pills to treat initial genital herpes infection.[7]

There were fifty patients involved in this study—thirty-five were women and fifteen were men. Each was suffering from an initial attack of genital herpes simplex. They were given either an acyclovir pill or a placebo ("sugar pill") five times a day for ten days. Each patient was examined carefully eight times during this period and then each month thereafter, looking for a recurrence of their genital disease. At the time these patients entered the study, they had had blisters for an average of three days. No patients had any herpes antibodies in their blood, indicating that this was a first infection for all of them. The acyclovir pill treatment markedly reduced the release of virus in all groups within three days, whereas those patients receiving placebo treatment continued to shed virus for an average of eleven days. Very few of the acyclovir patients developed new blisters after the third day, while nearly half of the placebo-treated patients continued to develop new sores. The acyclovir pills also enhanced the rapidity of healing of the genital ulcers in both men and women. All patients who received acyclovir treatment also had a marked shortening of the period in which they suffered pain, difficulty in urination, and general feelings of being ill.

Unfortunately, in the month of follow-up, there was no difference in the recurrence rate of genital herpes attacks between the group which had received acyclovir and the group which had received only placebo treatment. Nonetheless, the use of such pills may in the future shorten the period during which you are infectious, speed up your time of healing, prevent the development of new ulcers during an attack, and make you feel generally well sooner than if you received no therapy at all.

We can only hope that when all data from the studies now under way are finally compiled, the Food and Drug Administration will find sufficient evidence to justify approving additional uses of acyclovir such as those just described.

BVDU is the second of the new and highly specific antiherpes drugs which act only in virus-infected cells and leave your normal cells unscathed. BVDU has been found to be highly effective against herpes simplex virus type-1 and chicken pox-zoster virus. Unfortunately, it is only minimally effective against type-2 herpes. Nonetheless, it may prove highly useful, as one out of every three people under the age of twenty-four who have genital herpes have type-1 infections "below the waist."[87] This drug is currently under intensive investigation in Europe for the therapy of herpes infections of the eye, mouth, and widespread and local zoster (shingles) disease. In this country, many laboratory studies have been carried out, but the first of the human studies have yet to be initiated. An example of BVDU's great efficacy in severe herpes zoster disease is described in that section of this book.

The third major highly specific and nontoxic antiviral drug is called FIAC. This drug has been found to be highly effective against herpes simplex type-1 and type-2, as well as against herpes zoster virus. It is currently being tested intravenously in humans with widely spread and life-threatening herpes infections. Results of the early studies have been quite encouraging.

There are three additional antiviral drugs of current interest which are not members of the antimetabolite family. These are interferon, phosphonoformic acid (PFA), and 2-deoxy-D-glucose (2DG). None of these is yet commercially available, but you may have read or heard about them in the media.

Interferon is an antiviral protein produced naturally by the body when it is invaded by viruses or certain chemicals. When a virus enters a cell, the cell releases this protein so that neighboring cells can protect themselves from invasion by other viruses in the immediate tissue. In addition, interferon appears to increase the activity of the body's white blood cell, known as the natural killer cell. As we discussed earlier, the natural killer is a cell which immediately goes into action to defend the body against any foreign substance. It does not have to be programmed against that substance over a several-day period as do many of your other white cells, thereby delaying your body's defense against the infectious invasion. Interferon may also be produced in the laboratory by stimulating human or animal cells grown in tissue culture.

Until recently, this has been an extremely expensive and laborious process which has greatly limited the number of studies on the effect of interferon on human herpes infections. Many pharmaceutical companies with expertise in growing human cells for interferon production and in the science known as recombinant DNA, however, are now producing large quantities of interferon at relatively little cost. As these technologies are perfected, widespread studies will be carried out and the true place of interferon in the therapy of herpetic infections may be established. It is possible that the first submissions to the FDA for review of the interferon studies will come within the next two to three years. Current evidence indicates that interferon is effective in fighting herpes simplex infection of the eye and skin, as well as infections with herpes zoster. Perhaps of greater significance is the finding that interferon has an effect on fighting CMV infections. As noted in discussion of the previous antiviral drugs, these agents have little to no effect on CMV infections. Interferon may provide some help in the CMV epidemic, which is now quite active in the gay community.

PFA is found to be active against herpes type-1 infection, in that it shortens the time of healing sores on the skin. Unfortunately, this drug cannot be used internally because it builds up in your bones and the long-term effects of such a buildup are unknown. 2DG is a sugar-based drug which interferes with the manufacture of the protein coat surrounding herpetic chromosome. Without this protective coating, the virus is less infective. Preliminary tests treating women with genital herpes were encouraging, but these early promising results have yet to be proven conclusively. Both of these drugs need much more work done before we know their true value. As antiviral research is progressing now, however, it seems that they may never reach the levels of extended human study or FDA review for commercial release.

As the herpes viruses do not live in the skin but in the deep tissues such as the nerve cell ganglia or white blood cells, it makes sense that treatment with drugs such as ointments or drops will not prevent recurrences of herpetic disease. Use of these topical agents at best can only "cure" a current attack but can not reach the deep-seated virus reservoirs which lie beyond the reach of the antiviral drug. Even the administration of these drugs intravenously has been only transiently effective in suppressing the latent virus which lives in the deep tissues. This is probably because the latent form of most herpetic viruses is a chemical state which is not affected by our currently available antiviral medications.

Other forms of treatment have been mentioned throughout this book but despite early promise have failed to show meaningful therapeutic effect when more extensive studies were carried out in humans. Several of these are discussed in more detail under "Mouth and Skin Infections." The list of such doubtful, unsuccessful or, in some cases, dangerous therapies includes smallpox vaccination, dye-light therapy, levamisole enhancement of the blood immune defense systems, ether or chloroform mechanical rubbing of the blisters, vidarabine ointment on the skin, IDU ointment, or drops on the skin (DMSO with IDU may be one exception), BCG (bacille Calmette-Guérin) vaccine, type-1 or type-2 herpes simplex vaccine (Lupidon), L-lysine tablets, zinc sulfate ointment, and extract of seaweed. It is strongly recommended that should you be offered any of these therapies by a friend, acquaintance, or possibly even a physician, you question their use and seek a second opinion from a member of the medical profession.

Protecting Sexual Partners or Yourself from Infection

Other than treating your own acute attack to relieve symptoms, it is important to take steps to protect a sexual partner who may not have the infection or to protect yourself if your partner has it and you don't. The risk of catching herpes after a single sexual contact with an infected partner is not known, but more frequent contact with someone carrying genital herpes results in a greater than 50 percent chance of the virus spreading to you.

One key reason, beyond its currently incurable nature, that genital herpes is spreading so rapidly through the population is the development of the contraceptive pill, and contraceptives for insertion into the female womb (IUD, intrauterine device). Both of these lead to much less frequent use of the male condom ("safe" or "rubber") as a method of preventing pregnancy. The condom is an effective barrier which may protect a man from picking up herpes from his partner during intercourse or giving it to her or him during ejaculation. Any caring person with suspected genital herpes would be wise to use a condom when having sex with an uninfected partner.

Similarly, contraceptive foams or jellies, available without prescription at any drugstore, may be used to fill the vaginal canal and even smeared on the external genitalia before sexual activity. Such foams and jellies kill virus and will provide some, but not complete, protection against spreading venereal herpes during intercourse. The combination of a condom and contraceptive foam or jelly is obviously the best alternative of all.

Occasionally, it is wise to abstain from sexual activity altogether. The most obvious situation is when one partner has never had genital herpes and the other has obvious blisters or ulcers on the genitalia or rectum. Taking a cold shower and waiting a few days is well worth it for the uninfected partner or a partner whose herpes is not active. The last few weeks of pregnancy are another period during which sex should be avoided so that an otherwise quiet infection is not stirred up. This will be discussed further. Remember, herpes is most infectious during the blistering stage, least infectious (but still potentially infectious) during the crusted stage, but also contagious during the early numbness or tingling stages before the sores appear. *Don't take a chance; infectious virus may be present in recurrent herpes of the genitalia from the first warning symptoms and up to four to six days after the onset of recurrent symptoms.*

7. PREGNANCY, BIRTH, AND THE NEWBORN BABY

When we talk about herpes in connection with pregnancy and our babies, we are talking about something which must still be taken very seriously but with which the medical profession now has fairly extensive experience. With this experience has come knowledge of what to do and what not to do in assuring a happy outcome to your pregnancy, as well as the development of very good antiviral drugs should a problem develop despite all precaution. Even before we had much information on herpes in pregnancy, dangerous infections of mother or child were extremely rare; *only one to ten out of every ten thousand births* results in an infant who needs treatment for herpes. Significant infections, other than genital, in the mothers are rarer yet. In the discussion that follows, then, a wide variety of cases involving herpes and pregnancy are presented. *All are rare!* Some are presented to show you how well things can turn out with appropriate precautions and medical care, even when herpes enters the scene. Other cases are presented to show you what happened before we had the knowledge or therapy now available or what can happen if you do not take precautions during pregnancy and assure that you have regular obstetrical checkups for yourself and pediatric examinations for your baby. *Every complication discussed here could have been prevented or, if it had happened more recently, been successfully treated.*

Pregnancy

When genital herpes and pregnancy come at the same time, each can make the other worse and more complicated. It is generally felt that if a woman does develop the disease while carrying a child, the infection will be much more severe than if she were not pregnant. As a result, some of the most difficult cases of venereal or other forms of herpes seen are those in pregnant women. The effect of active or even silent virus infection during the first few months of pregnancy are not well known, but there is some evidence that a bad attack may cause a miscarriage or excessive weight loss in the infant. There is little evidence, however, that, short of direct infection in the womb, herpes causes congenital birth defects.

First Genital Infection

A first genital infection during pregnancy poses a much greater threat to your baby than recurrent disease. In a first infection, you have no body defenses (antiherpes antibodies and white cells) ready to control the process. This allows much more virus to grow and spread and the infection to last much longer. In addition, your baby may not have any antibodies to fight herpes. Unborn babies normally receive antibodies against many viruses and bacteria from their mother's blood across the placenta (afterbirth). It takes about ten days for antibodies to develop once an infection has occurred. Therefore, if you have your first genital herpes infection several weeks (or years) before delivery, both you and your baby will have at least the partial protection antibodies provide. If, however, you develop the infection within ten days of delivery, you and the baby will have very low levels of protective antibodies. In addition, there is a greatly increased risk that your baby will be exposed directly to high levels of herpes virus if delivery is through the birth canal.

Recurrent Genital Infections

The risks to the baby are less in recurrent attacks because the infection is less severe and antiherpes antibodies will provide some protection to your baby. Unfortunately, it may be very difficult for your doctor to tell whether your infection is first or recurrent, as the diseases can look alike. To complicate matters, in more than half of the babies born with herpes infections, their mothers had silent, unnoticed attacks of genital herpes at the time of delivery. This is why a close watch by your obstetrician and appropriate *Pap smears are so critical* throughout your pregnancy. Checkups will make you feel better, reassured, and greatly help to avoid any unnecessary complications during or after your pregnancy. The following case is an example of the *tragic results which may come from not seeing your physician regularly during your pregnancy,* not informing him of possible infectious complications, or delaying cesarean section in the presence of ruptured membranes.[18]

A seventeen-year-old woman was first seen when she was six months into her pregnancy. Prenatal records were completed and laboratory studies ordered by paramedical personnel, but the mother failed to keep any of her appointments with her physician. During her pregnancy, she was seen at a routine outpatient clinic for some form of urinary tract infection (herpes?) and a mild upper-respiratory infection. She went into *premature labor* at eight months and *was only then seen by a doctor for the first time in her entire pregnancy.* At that time, she had a fever of 101° F, the cause of which could not be determined. Her membranes had ruptured prematurely and she underwent several vaginal examinations during the twelve hours of observation before a cesarean section was performed because there was no progression of labor. The mother's fever resolved and she remained normal throughout the hospital stay. The four-pound male baby was admitted from the delivery room to the intermediate intensive care nursery, where examination revealed only prematurity. An intensive work-up was done, however, because the mother had received antibiotics for fever of unknown cause. The child remained normal until the fifth day, when he suddenly developed a fever of 105° F and yellow blisters developed on his scalp. Herpes simplex was diagnosed and his condition deteriorated rapidly. He was given two intensive courses of the systemic antiviral drug, vidarabine. Despite all supportive therapy, however, the baby died on the seventh day of life. Cultures were all positive for herpes type-2.

Because of the infant's illness, a repeat pelvic exam was performed on the mother. She appeared entirely normal. However, a virus culture of her cervix was positive for herpes simplex type-2.

The preceding tragedy might well have been avoided had this mother kept her appointments with her physician, informed him when she was having urinary tract difficulties, and, if known, given him a history that she might have had genital herpes in the past.

Herpes Infections in Pregnant Women

As we shall discuss further, herpes simplex type-1 or -2 infections during pregnancy may or may not have bad effects on the newborn infant. But there is another person to be considered during this period, and that is the effect of herpes on you, the mother. As noted, it is well known that if a genital herpes infection develops during pregnancy, it will be much more severe than if you were not pregnant. Fortunately, more serious forms of herpes are extremely rare, but early recognition of the symptoms is essential, as we now have treatment more effective than that available in the past. The following case reports have been put in to illustrate the different outcomes which may occur when a mother develops a herpes infection of her brain while she is pregnant and what effect this may have, not only on her but on her baby.[27]

This twenty-three-year-old woman was three months pregnant when she first saw her physician for complaints of back pain and temperatures up to 103° F. All studies were normal and she was placed on antibiotics. Six days later, she was seen with a temperature of 103° F and appeared quite sleepy. She was admitted to the hospital with a presumptive diagnosis of encephalitis (brain infection) and consultations with a neurologist and internist were obtained.

She complained of a throbbing headache that was made worse by movement or bright light. She denied other visual disturbances or a stiff neck. On examination, she was extremely sleepy and had a high fever and rapid pulse. Blood pressure was normal and the physical and neurological examination was normal. A spinal fluid tap indicated viral inflammation of the brain and spinal cord, but viral cultures were reported as negative. During the ensuing days, she became worse, occasionally lapsing into coma or hallucinating, but, without any specific therapy, gradually began to improve spontaneously. She was ultimately discharged just three weeks after admission.

During her hospital stay, doctors discussed with her the possibility of bad effects of her illness on her unborn child and offered her an abortion if she wished it. She stated that she would not consider an abortion under any circumstances.

The remainder of her pregnancy was normal and she was admitted at term in active labor. Seven hours later, she was delivered of a seven-pound male baby who was perfectly normal on examination. The baby has been followed for four years and has developed normally both physically and mentally. The patient has also been carefully followed and has no neurological damage.

Author's comment: The key weakness in this report is that herpes virus was not conclusively proven to be the cause of the brain infection.

This second case is another illustration of proven severe herpetic illness in a pregnant woman with an ultimate good result, both for her and her baby.[50]

A twenty-one-year-old woman was in the ninth month of her first pregnancy when she developed fever, vomiting, and pain on urination. She deined prior oral or genital herpes, but examination revealed that her external genitalia were swollen and painful, the cervix was inflamed, and she had diffuse tenderness of her abdomen. A Pap stain of the cervical smear was consistent with herpes simplex infection.

Her temperature persisted and a diagnosis of disseminated herpes infection was considered. On the third day, a live and completely healthy six-pound baby girl was delivered by cesarean section. At the time of surgery, the mother's stomach area was explored. It was found that her liver and pancreas were diffusely involved with inflamed lesions and there was an abnormal amount of fluid present.

After delivery, the patient's fever cleared, but on the third postoperative day she complained of headache, became very sleepy and disoriented, and had five convulsions. Spinal tap and electronic diagnostic tests were consistent with a diagnosis of herpes encephalitis (brain infection) and intravenous therapy with the antiviral drug, vidarabine, was begun. Three days later, she was more alert but still suffered from headache and pain in the abdomen. There was continued evidence of liver damage and her heart rate slowed. After five days, the dosage of vidarabine was decreased and therapy was discontinued two days later.

Her pancreas and liver infection and cardiac disease gradually resolved over the next ten days. Repeat brain tests showed only minimal abnormality and she went home in good condition on her thirty-first hospital day.

Since that time, she has had no recurrence of fever, convulsions, blisters, or genital disease. She has occasional episodes of dizziness and moderately severe memory loss but otherwise lives a normal life. Her infant daughter never demonstrated evidence of involvement with herpes and has undergone normal growth and development.

Viral cultures of the liver confirmed that this was a herpes simplex type-2 infection. Blood tests for antibody levels revealed that this was a primary infection with type-2 virus and that the patient had never been infected with type-1 herpes. She, therefore, had no preexisting antibodies to any herpes virus which might have made her disease less severe.

The foregoing cases of severe herpes infections in pregnant women had fortunate outcomes for mother and baby alike. Unfortunately, in a few rare instances, this was not always so. If there is one thing that we may learn from the case described above, and from the case above where an antiviral drug was used, it is that if antiviral therapy is to work at all, it must be given very early in the course of infection. This means that it is very important for you to notify your doctor at once should you suspect some of the early signs which indicate that you may be developing active herpes infection.

Detecting Genital Herpes Near the Time of Delivery

Not every pregnancy can or should be watched with diagnostic Pap smears or virus cultures, as it is best to avoid scraping the cervix and birth canal in totally normal, unthreatened situations. You should help your doctor in making decisions about whether to do Pap smears near delivery time by telling him if:

1. you have ever had genital herpes in the past;
2. you had genital herpes at any time during your present pregnancy (if your doctor does not already know about it);
3. you have had herpes outside the genital area but below your waist or on your fingers, as this may mean there is genital infection as well;
4. you have had sexual intercourse with someone with known genital herpes.

Purpose of the Pap or Tzanck Smear

Taking Pap or Tzanck smears to test for the presence of *active or silent infectious herpes* in the birth canal is done because your doctor must decide whether your baby should be allowed to pass through the birth canal or be delivered by cesarean section (through a surgical opening in your abdomen). If there is no evidence of virus near the time of birth, the risk to the baby is very very small. Almost every case of herpes in newborn babies was picked up either during passage through an actively or silently infected canal or by the virus climbing up to the baby from an infected canal if the waters (membranes) had broken several hours before delivery took place. Although there is little question that cesarean section is somewhat harder on the mother for a day or two after delivery, the actual risks associated with the surgery are minimal and will greatly help to protect your baby from herpetic infection if there is evidence of virus in your birth canal.

Who Should Have a Cesarean Section?

Herpes infections can be so destructive to an infant (who could be normal if cesarean section is performed), it is now generally recommended that this surgery be done if you have a definite first infection genital herpes near the end of your pregnancy. This is only if your waters have not broken or have been broken less than six hours before your baby is to be delivered. Your doctor must also feel that you can safely undergo the operation. If your waters have been broken more than six hours, the virus has already had time to reach your baby and your doctor may decide to allow the infant to pass through the birth canal.

There is no definite policy concerning cesarean section if you are found to have *recurrent* active or silent infection at the time of delivery. There are, however, some very good reasons for you to discuss having a cesarean section with your doctor. These include:

1. the uncertainty of always being able to tell a first infection from a recurrent one or a reinfection with a new herpes virus;

2. the generally excellent outcome of cesarean section for both you and your baby;
3. the potentially severe effect of herpes on your baby if it does pick up the virus;
4. the sorrowful effects such an illness would have on you and your family;
5. the unknown long-term effects on your baby if it develops a silent congenital infection.

The decision may be difficult for you and your doctor, but you must take into account all of these factors. You must do what is best for you and your baby within the limits of today's knowledge.

Amniocentesis (Testing Fluid From the Womb Before Birth)

Unfortunately, although cesarean section is the best procedure in most cases, it cannot be 100 percent guaranteed that your baby will not contract herpes. There is some evidence that, in rare instances, the virus can spread across the placenta before the waters break or labor begins. If you have a first or active infection near delivery time, your doctor may want to perform a procedure called amniocentesis. This procedure causes little discomfort. It involves passing a small needle through your abdominal wall into the womb to draw off a small sample of the fluid and loose cells in which your baby is floating. Examination of the cells for evidence of virus is helpful, but your doctor will not totally rely on it for decision making. Only actual culturing of herpes virus from this fluid is a reliable indication that your infant already has the infection. If virus is present, your doctor may decide to let your baby come through the birth canal unless cesarean section is needed for other reasons. If no virus is found in the fluid, your doctor will probably perform a cesarean section if there is active herpes in the birth canal, thus protecting your child from being exposed to the infected tissues.

The following case report is presented to show that while amniocentesis can be a critical test in deciding whether to have your baby through the birth canal or by cesarean section, actual recovery of herpes virus from the fluid is by far the most reliable part of the test. *Abnormal cell changes alone do not necessarily indicate that the virus has infected the womb or the baby.*[4]

The patient was a twenty-nine-year-old woman who had had two previous unexpected miscarriages. Examination revealed that she had a weak cervix (womb opening) and a surgical procedure to hold it closed during her pregnancy was performed. She did well throughout her pregnancy until approximately three weeks before her due date. At this time, blisters appeared on her external genitalia and were found to be due to herpes simplex virus. An amniocentesis was performed one week later for both examination of cellular material and virus culture. Examination of cells from the infant showed changes typical of herpes infection. It was assumed, therefore, that the child was already infected with herpes and should be allowed to pass through the birth canal, despite the presence of active infection of his mother's genitalia. Seven days after the amniocentesis, however, the virus cultures were recorded as negative and the decision to allow vaginal delivery was reversed. A cesarean section was performed and a healthy seven-pound male infant was delivered two days before the estimated due date. Both the mother and infant were isolated and observed for ten days. Multiple virus cultures were taken from the amniotic fluid and the infant's urine, throat, and spinal fluid—and all were negative. The newborn was healthy and without evidence of herpetic infection at the three-month follow-up examination.

The above case demonstrates how important it is to have all information at hand before decisions concerning delivery are made. In this case, it was assumed for a full week that the unborn infant was already infected with herpes virus. It is difficult to imagine how stressful this must have been, both to the parents and to the physician in charge of making decisions for the benefit of both mother and child. Once all the information, including the virus cultures, was in, however, the entire situation changed and the outcome, in this case, was a happy one.

Sexual Intercourse During Pregnancy

The effect of sexual intercourse on an established pregnancy may pose a problem for many couples if herpes has entered the picture. During the first seven or eight months of pregnancy, sexual activity should cause little difficulty, even if the mother temporarily reactivates genital herpes. If, however, she has never had genital herpes and her sexual partner is known to have it, it would be most advisable that condoms and contraceptive foams or jellies be used for their antiviral properties throughout the pregnancy. This will give at least some partial protection to the mother against getting herpes in the birth canal. Sexual activity should be avoided at any time one partner has known active disease. Intercourse may be resumed once the attack has passed.

The risks of picking up type-1 herpes in the genital area during oral-genital sex should not be forgotten and this activity should be avoided if one partner has a cold sore around the mouth or nose. Type-1 herpes can cause just as dangerous genital infections as type-2.

Toward the end of pregnancy, particularly during the last month, it is best not to have any sexual intercourse because of the increased risk of reactivating disease after intercourse and because premature birth is not uncommon in women with genital herpes. If it is absolutely not possible to avoid sexual contact late in pregnancy, the usual precautions of condoms, contraceptive foams or jellies, and good hygiene—with soap and warm water bathing—is recommended. Vaginal douching should never be performed without the advice and consent of your doctor.

The following case demonstrates the importance of *avoiding sexual intercourse during the last few days before delivery* of your baby if either you or your partner is known to have genital herpes. It is also an example of the extreme importance of telling your doctor if you even suspect that one of you may have a genital infection, as this entire tragedy could have been prevented.[44]

This twenty-one-year-old woman had undergone a perfectly normal pregnancy and when, at midnight, she ruptured her membranes on her due date, she immediately sought medical care and was delivered of her third child, a normal baby, three hours later. Delivery was through the vagina and the postpartum period was normal. The baby and mother went home on the third day after delivery.

When the baby was eleven days old, the mother noted that the infant was constantly drowsy and not eating well. She brought the baby to the hospital and the child was admitted. On the second day in the hospital, a small blister was discovered on the head, but no others were found. A Tzanck staining from scraping of the ulcer and virus cultures revealed that the baby had a herpes simplex virus infection. Intravenous therapy with the antiviral drug, vidarabine, was begun, but the baby's condition worsened rapidly over the ensuing days and the infant died at three weeks of age from widespread herpes type-2 infection.

Further questioning of the patient revealed that although she had no signs of herpes infection at or near the time of delivery, she had had sexual intercourse on the night prior to delivery. At this time, they had noticed that her husband had a tender blister on his penis. He had had these blisters on several occasions throughout the previous month and they had been disregarded by both the patient and her husband. She did not tell her obstetrician about these sores, but the subsequent evaluation of her husband's ulcer after the baby's death revealed that he was intermittently infected by recurrent herpes simplex virus type-2 on his penis.

This tragic outcome of an otherwise normal pregnancy can only serve to emphasize how important it is for you to tell your doctor anything that you may notice or that may cause you concern, no matter how trivial it may seem at the time. It is important for you to *tell your doctor both your own history of any genital infections and to tell him if your sexual partner may have had such an infection.* This will obviously change your doctor's management of your pregnancy and delivery and he or she will remind you of the importance of avoiding sexual intercourse, if possible, during the last four weeks before you expect the birth of your baby.

8. HERPES IN THE NEWBORN CHILD

Watching the New Baby for Herpes

Although the parents may have taken all precautions, newborn infants of parents with herpes should be watched carefully for signs of the disease. If your baby has been infected at the time of birth, the disease will develop in two to twelve days. If a herpes infection starts after that time, your baby probably caught it after birth from someone with a cold sore or other active herpes. Signs that your baby may be developing herpes include unusual sleepiness, fever, redness or irritation of the eyes, and blisters on the skin or lips or inside the mouth. Ophthalmologists (eye physicians) as well as pediatricians may be asked to examine your infant.

As many infants born to infected mothers have little or no blood antibodies to fight the herpes virus, your doctor may decide to give your baby an injection of gamma globulin as a precaution. Most lots of this material contain high levels of antibodies against both type-1 and type-2 herpes. This will temporarily help to protect your child.

Discharge from the hospital need not be delayed for an apparently healthy infant, but you should return the baby to your doctor immediately as a true emergency if any of the signs or symptoms mentioned above or convulsions (seizures or fits) occur. Your baby should be re-examined by your doctor within a few days of discharge, in any event, regardless of how well it looks.

If your baby develops herpes, it will not take long before the true severity of the infection becomes apparent. Many infants will develop blisters or ulcers of the skin or mouth and be unable to feed. Their eyes may become red and ulcerated with watery discharge, in which case the infant may bury his or her head in the mattress to avoid the irritation of light. More severe symptoms may develop within a matter of hours or a day or two and include fever, loss of appetite, yellow and/or blue discoloration of the skin and lips, and cramps. The main body organs involved are 1) the liver (in viral hepatitis), which leads to bleeding and jaundice (yellow discoloration of the skin and eyes) and 2) the brain, which causes sleepiness, convulsions, and coma. Both forms can cause death in more than half the babies affected and the survivors are usually severely retarded for life. For about one out of every ten infants with herpes, the disease remains localized to the skin or eyes and the children do well. It is fortunate that *congenital herpes occurs in only about one to ten out of every ten thousand births.*

Diagnosis

Diagnosis should be made as rapidly as possible, so that treatment may be started immediately. Herpes in a newborn may be diagnosed on the basis of skin, eye, or mouth blisters alone, or may require putting a tube down the baby's esophagus (the canal leading from mouth to stomach) for biopsy and culture—or the taking of a brain biopsy and culture. About one quarter of all herpes in the newborn is due to type-1, the remainder to type-2, but either type may produce equally severe illness.

Treatment

Unlike many forms of herpes, specific therapy for herpes of the brain is now commercially available. Vidarabine or acyclovir,* if given in the veins very early after the onset of disease, are effective drugs both in preventing death and in reducing severe side effects from the disease. The longer therapy is delayed, the greater the chance of death and the less the drug effect on preventing serious damage to the brain. Vidarabine, of course, has some side effects itself, but these are largely reversible and certainly less than those caused by the disease. Herpes of the eyes may be safely treated with antiviral ointments or eye drops and is discussed later.

Beyond specific antiviral treatment, there is little your doctor can do for an infant with widespread herpes except supportive

* Acyclovir is not yet FDA-approved for use in brain infections.

therapy in the form of intravenous fluids, antiseizure drugs, reducing fever, and hoping that the disease will run its course in a mild and nondestructive path.

Once your infant gets *beyond the newborn period,* a few months of age, if exposure to herpes occurs it will generally result in *illness no worse than that seen in older children or adults.* Ninety-five percent of these first infections produce no visible illness (see "Mouth and Skin Infections").

Case Reports of Herpes-Infected Newborns

When an infant contracts herpes infection while still in his mother's uterus, the disease may be either local or widespread. Local infections may be found in the eye, skin, mouth, or the brain. These infections are *extremely rare* but may be due either to type-1 or type-2 herpes, as the virus has spread through the mother's bloodstream and across the placenta to the baby from some other site in her body, such as her mouth or her genitalia. The following is a case report of twin infants who acquired herpes infection while in their mother's uterus. It is included to show that such an infection can be local and amenable to treatment with a good outcome.[22]

A seventeen-year-old mother was delivered of two male infants by cesarean section without previous rupture of her membranes. Her pregnancy had been uncomplicated, except for a brief flulike infection at seven months. Neither parent had a history of genital herpes. Examination of the first twin immediately after birth was normal, except for his left eye which was red and clouded in the normally clear central window, the cornea. He was found to have a herpes ulcer at this site. Examination of his brother was entirely normal. By the next day, the clouding and redness of the first twin's eye had become worse and, despite antibiotic therapy, he continued to have more severe disease in his eye. On the fifth day, virus cultures and scrapings were taken and indicated a herpetic lesion. Antiviral therapy with IDU (idoxuridine) was begun, but there was little therapeutic response until the IDU was discontinued and the patient treated with vidarabine ointment, which resulted in significant improvement within a few days.

During the second week after birth, the second twin developed blisters on his right lid but no direct involvement of his eye. He was treated with IDU and the eye did not become involved with viral infection.

Because the doctors were concerned that the virus infection might spread in both children, they were treated prophylactically with intravenous vidarabine for ten days. Virus cultures from the first twin's eye had grown out herpes simplex type-1. Cultures taken from his mother's cervix one week after the delivery were negative.

At the time of discharge from the hospital, both children were in excellent health, although the first twin had some scarring of his left eye.

The above case is important because it demonstrates that infants may be infected with herpes while still in their mother's womb and yet not develop a widely spread or fatal infection. As this mother's membranes had not broken at the time of her cesarean section, it seems clear that the spread of virus was through the blood from some other site in the body. Because this was type-1 herpes, it is likely that this came from an infection around her mouth and may possibly have been the cause of her fever and illness during the seventh month of her pregnancy.

Unfortunately, not all herpes infection of infants still in the womb are as benign as this one.

Herpes infection in new babies, while very rare, is an extremely serious illness. Nonetheless, as noted above, as our therapy for this disease becomes better with the development of new and better drugs such as vidarabine and acyclovir, more and more babies may be expected to survive. In addition, *herpes in a new baby is not always a disaster*. The following are three case reports of infants who were born with herpes infections and who not only survived but who, by and large, did well during a period when we had absolutely no antiviral therapy to offer them. As you will see, the only adverse effects are that one baby developed more slowly than normal and that all three went through a period of having recurrent infections for several months after the initial disease.[21]

Case 1: A four-pound female baby was born prematurely after a pregnancy complicated only by mild intermittent vaginal bleeding during the month prior to delivery. Examination in the delivery room revealed small red patches on both sides of the baby's face, neck, and on the right shoulder. These were about one-half inch in diameter, circular, slightly depressed, and reddened. Six days later, blisters appeared in these areas and on the right wrist and back. Herpes simplex was isolated from these blisters, but blood, urine, and stool cultures were negative. By two weeks of life, the ulcers had dried and crusted and they had almost completely cleared by the third week of life. At no time during the hospitalization did the baby appear ill.

During the ensuing eight months, the baby developed crops of blisters every three to four weeks in the areas which had been involved at the time of birth. These blisters would heal and clear within two days. In addition, she developed blisters on her abdomen, which had not previously been involved. She gained weight normally and had no obvious abnormal physical or neurologic problem. However, developmental testing indicated that she was functioning at a three-month level when she was fourteen months of age. All chemical and electrographic studies of her brain were normal at this time.

Case 2: A five-pound female baby was the first child born to a nineteen-year-old woman after ten hours of uncomplicated labor. The only abnormality noted during her pregnancy was a white vaginal discharge without itching during the last few weeks before delivery. No sores were noticed on the external genitalia at delivery or during the several days after birth.

The baby was entirely normal at birth, with the exception of flat red sores on the face, chest, and back. She did well in the nursery and was sent home on the second day of life. During the next three days, the baby developed blisters in these reddened areas but had no fever and was eating well.

The baby was admitted to the hospital when she was seven days of age because of numerous small groups of blisters in the areas of redness noted at birth. Vesicles were also found on the right side of the abdomen and right arm. Herpes simplex virus was cultured from the blisters present on the baby when she was nine days of age. All the blisters were drying by the thirteenth day of age without any specific therapy and the baby was sent home.

During the first eighteen months of her life, the infant had several similar recurrences of blisters in the previously involved area. However, the baby's growth and development were entirely normal.

Case 3: A six-pound male baby was the second child born to an eighteen-year-old woman at full term. The mother had noticed vaginal pain and burning a few days before delivery. At the time of birth, there were no signs or symptoms suggesting herpetic disease. The baby was delivered by cesarean section because of poor progression of labor. The membranes had been ruptured for sixteen hours before delivery.

The baby was taken to the nursery, where a boggy swelling was noted on the top of his head. By the time he was five days old, the swelling had cleared, but two discrete crusted areas were present. On the seventh day, a two-inch bloody crust appeared in this area, surrounded by many blisters. Two days later, blisters appeared behind the left ear and left upper arm and wrist. Cultures taken from these blisters were positive for herpes simplex virus. All blisters followed a similar course and were completely healed by two weeks time. The infant remained well and had no fever throughout his hospital course. He was sent home on his eighteenth day of life.

During the following sixteen months of observation, the infant had a total of six recurrences of blisters at various sites on his body, including the scalp, elbow, ear, and wrist, all of which cleared without treatment within two to four days. His growth and development was normal throughout the periods of observation.

These three cases are most encouraging in terms of herpes in the newborn not always being a severe and fatal disease. Nonetheless, one of the babies involved did have slower than normal development.

It is possible that herpes infection contracted by a fetus or newborn child is a very rare cause of physical or mental retardation, which may not be noted until later in life. Because two of these babies were born with herpes already present, we must assume that the infection took place *in utero,* possibly by passage of the virus across the placenta. The third baby, the one delivered by cesarean section, may have acquired his virus by the germ climbing from the cervix through the ruptured membranes and into the area where the baby was located. We can also learn from these cases that although cesarean section will greatly reduce the chance of a baby contracting herpes in the presence of active infection in the mother, it is no guarantee that a child cannot become infected in the womb. Similarly, these cases should alert all physicians to the fact that herpes infection of newborn babies may not always be fatal but may establish itself as a recurrent illness in an otherwise normal child. *These recurrences, when and if they come, are no different or more severe in a basically healthy child than those seen with routine cold sores in an adult.*

9. PRECAUTIONS AFTER BIRTH

Prevention of Infection After Delivery If Genital Herpes Is Active

If you did not have active genital herpes or other active herpes, such as a cold sore at the time of delivery, no special precautions are necessary. As long as your infection is inactive and no virus is present, your baby is not at risk. If, however, your doctor feels that your herpes was active at the time of delivery, he or she may wish to put you in a private room to protect other mothers and their babies. Everyone in contact with you may be asked to use gowns and gloves and all materials, such as bed linens and dressings covering your genital area, will be specially handled and be disposed of with great care.

You may be allowed to handle your infant if it is healthy—but under supervised conditions. You must thoroughly wash your hands before touching the baby. You may be asked to sit in a chair away from your bed and to wear a clean gown and gloves. Once your baby has been with you, even under such careful circumstances, the child may be treated as potentially infected with herpes and kept away from the other babies in the nursery. Do not feel that because your baby is kept separate from the others this means it is infected.

A good example of what can happen *if such precautions are not taken* by hospital personnel occurred when three babies, two of them twins, were born within four days of each other in the same hospital.[17] Four days after birth, the first child developed fever, became very sleepy, began to vomit, and to have diarrhea. One day later, the twins were born and four days later began to have difficulty breathing. One twin went into shock and died within twenty-four hours of the onset of her disease; the second twin died similarly the next day. The child who was vomiting finally went into coma and died three days after the second twin was lost. Both mothers were found by blood test to have had type-2 herpes infection at the time of delivery.

This was a true tragedy for these infants born with congenital herpes, but an almost unspeakable tragedy was occurring at the same time and may well have been prevented. A perfectly healthy one-month-old baby was brought from another hospital into the same hospital nursery for evaluation of a harmless heart murmur. It was during the same period that the first three babies were isolated in separate rooms next door. Fourteen days later, the fourth baby suddenly became sleepy and began to have convulsions. A rash of blisters appeared over her right cheek, arms, and chest. She went into continuous seizure activity and died within ten days of the onset of symptoms. This child's mother had no evidence of any herpes on exam, by history, or by blood tests. The source of virus in this last sorrowful death was felt to be through some herpes-infected object or person in contact both with the three infected babies and the initially healthy infant as she was rocked and fed in the general hallway outside the isolation rooms. A sad lesson, indeed, but one which emphasizes the need for the greatest precaution where congenital herpes is concerned.

Precautions If Nongenital Herpes Is Active

Genital herpes is, however, not the only form of this viral disease which threatens newborns. There is much evidence showing that type-1 herpes is just as dangerous to a new baby as type-2. *If you have active nongenital herpes, such as a cold sore on your lips or skin,* your doctor may feel that precautions similar to those taken for women with active genital infections should be taken. As blisters are more infectious than sores in the crusted stage, steps may be taken in an attempt to speed up clearing of the herpes so that you may be safely united with your new baby. These steps include drying treatment such as previously mentioned, or twice-daily painting of the sores with any of a number of drying/antiseptic medications, such as povidone-iodine or tincture of benzoin. The ulcers will crust within two or three days and your doctor may then allow you to have your baby, but you may still have to wear a fresh gown and gloves. In addition, you may have to wear a mask or dressing over the herpetic sores until they have totally healed.

Mothers with either active genital or nongenital herpes may, with the doctor's permission, visit their babies in the nursery if the child is not allowed out to the mother's room. This means using the same gown-glove precautions previously outlined. The baby may be kept separate from the others or in a special care unit just before and once contact with you has been made. All this precaution may make you feel as if you are a carrier of some dreadful disease, but the prevention of such tragedies as the four babies who died from herpes is well worth a few days of inconvenience.

The following case report is another excellent example of why you, as a new mother, must take extreme precaution in the management and observation of your baby if you yourself have herpes active anywhere in your body, type-1 or type-2.[29]

A young woman had been admitted to the hospital for fever and sore throat. She did, in fact, have inflamed tonsils, on which many small ulcers were noticed. In addition, she had cold sores around her mouth. There was no evidence of genital herpes, however.

The next day, she delivered a normal five-pound baby girl. While in the hospital, the baby showed no signs of illness and was breast fed by her mother *without precaution against herpes being taken*. One week later, on the day of discharge from the hospital, the baby was found to have a conjunctivitis in the left eye. An antibiotic was instilled.

The next day, the mother called her own doctor and they agreed that the eye treatment should be continued. That evening the doctor visited the home and found the baby to be in good condition other than the red eye. A few hours later, the baby had a brief attack of cramps and the mother tried unsuccessfully to take its temperature. The doctor was called again.

Examination revealed that the baby had widely spread herpes simplex infection.

This case, while very rare, is important because it demonstrates not only the rapidity with which herpesvirus can cause severe illness in a new baby, but also the importance of taking every precaution against herpes when the mother, or anyone contacting the baby, has type-1, just as you would every precaution if type-2 were active.

When Can I Hold My Baby Without All These Precautions?

At this point, you may be asking yourself: "If I have herpes, can I ever safely cuddle my child?" The answer is an unequivocal yes. As you know, in a basically healthy person, herpes infections last less than a week unless the episode is a primary one. In the study cited earlier under acyclovir in "Therapy and Prevention of Genital Herpes" the longest duration of virus-shedding (the contagious period) was only seven days and that was in untreated primary infections. This should give you some idea of the length of time when it is possible for you to pass the virus on. The same length of time or shorter applies to oral cold sores or other herpes ulcers of your skin.

This means that within a few days of coming home after a few days' hospital stay you will be noninfectious and may handle and love your baby just as any mother may and should. *Ask your doctor or pediatrician just when it is safe to stop glove, mask or other precaution. Handwashing and general good body hygiene,* including washing your breasts before each feeding, if you have elected to breast feed, *is always important regardless of whether you have had herpes.*

What about friends and herpes? You can't really ask everyone if he or she had genital herpes before allowing them near your baby. It is unlikely that anyone with active genital herpes would ask to hold the baby anyway but for those instances where you just don't know, make it a general rule that everyone washes his or her hands well with warm water and soap before picking up the infant. For friends and relatives with cold sores of the mouth or face, the rules are a bit different. You can see that there is activity. In this case, a polite but firm request that they not handle the baby until their sores have healed should suffice. It is no different from asking someone with an ordinary head cold not to hold the baby until the infection is gone. They will certainly understand your request.

Rooming-In (Having Your New Baby Live in Your Hospital Room)

Rooming-in on a continuous basis has clear advantages as well as disadvantages where genital herpes is involved. If your baby stays in your room and is cared for by you at all times, there is less chance of introducing herpes into the general nursery and less contact between the potentially infected baby and the hospital staff. Rooming-in establishes an early close contact between you and your infant and helps to prepare you for care of the baby once at home. But if you have active herpes anywhere on your body, continuous rooming-in is wise only when there are enough hospital nurses and aides available to help you and supervise you carefully to be sure that you carry out all necessary precautions to protect your baby. In large city hospitals, this is often not possible. In this case, the infant is usually left mainly in the nursery and intermittent rooming-in undertaken at planned times, such as for feeding, and only when personnel are available to train you in appropriate precautions. This will minimize any risk to your baby.

Breast Feeding

Breast feeding is often an area of great concern to mothers with active or quiet herpes infections of any type. The following case is so rare that it is presented only because there is a perfectly feasible alternate reason as to why this baby came down with herpes —not because of breast feeding. As the case is known to some doctors, however, it needs further discussion.[13]

This male infant was born through the vaginal canal after a full-term, uncomplicated pregnancy. On the sixth day of life, he developed hoarseness which progressed to an inability to utter any sound at all. Examination revealed many blisters on the roof of his mouth and the back of his throat. Virus cultures were positive for herpes simplex type-1. All other tests, including spinal fluid examination, were normal.

Two days later, the baby was hospitalized with a cluster of herpes blisters on the front of his chest. Three days later, he became sleepy and had the onset of focal convulsions that were not well controlled with drugs. Spinal fluid examination was abnormal and, because herpes encephalitis was suspected, treatment with vidarabine was begun and continued for ten days. Over the next ten days, his sleepiness improved and seizures stopped and he began to feed normally.

Because the infant had developed herpes shortly after his birth, his mother underwent a thorough evaluation in an attempt to locate the source of the virus. Virus cultures from her cervix, vagina, and throat, taken fourteen days after delivery, were negative. Cultures of her breast milk, taken nine days after delivery, however, were positive for herpes simplex type-1. No blisters or other abnormalities were found on examination of his mother's breast. Cultures from the infant's throat were also positive for herpes simplex type-1.

It is certainly recognized that cytomegalovirus (CMV), another member of the herpes virus family, is passed from mother to child through the breast milk. Because CMV appears to be passed together with specific antibodies, the baby is rendered somewhat immune to the virus and may not develop overt infection. As discussed in the section "The Gay Population and Herpes Infections," the CMV virus may present itself later in life in a very worrisome fashion.

The passage of herpes simplex virus through breast milk, however, is not a well-recognized phenomenon and has been questioned by other members of the medical community. Specific criticisms against the above described case are that the mother may well have had an inapparent genital herpes infection with type-1. The fact that her virus cultures from the genital area were negative at fourteen days after birth did not mean that she was not shedding virus at the time the baby was delivered. It is possible that the child picked up type-1 herpes from his mother's birth canal, developed sores in his own mouth, and then inoculated his mother's nipples during early breast feeding. This is an entirely believable course of events and, until further studies are done, we must hold our judgment on the passage of herpes simplex via breast milk in abeyance. Certainly there is no reason for a mother with a history of herpes to avoid breast feeding unless her physician feels there is some valid reason to do so—e.g., active infection elsewhere in her body. When you consider that since time immemorial millions upon millions of women with herpes have breast fed their children without any problems, worrying about breast feeding your own child should not be a concern in the absence of active genital or oral infection.

10. CANCER AND HERPES

Viruses from the herpes family have definitely been shown to cause cancer in certain animals. This, of course, makes all herpes viruses suspect of causing this disease in humans. Two such viruses have been associated with causing a form of lymphoma (related to Hodgkin's disease) and to cancer of the throat. There have also been a few reports of cancers arising on the lips of patients at the site of recurring herpes infections, but there is no really good evidence that these two are related. The relationship between herpes type-2, cytomegalovirus and a cancer called Kaposi's sarcoma is discussed under "The Gay Population and Herpetic Infections."

Cervical Cancer (Internal Genital Cancer)

Of great concern today is the increasing evidence that genital herpes may cause malignant disease in women. Ten years have passed since it was first suggested that there may be a connection between cancer of the female cervix (vaginal end of the womb) and herpes type-2. Certainly, it has now been shown that women with chronic genital herpes or high type-2 antibodies in their blood have a greater chance of developing cancer of the cervix than women who do not have this infection. It has also been shown that type-2 herpes can cause early cancerlike changes in animals. But the isolation of herpes from a cancer does not necessarily mean that the virus caused it. It appears that type-2 herpes is but one of many factors that must be present for cancer to develop. Other associated factors, demonstrated in several studies, include a number of activities which may come as a surprise to many people. Some of them we can have control over; others we can not. Such factors are: 1) marriage; 2) broken marriage; 3) multiple marriages; 4) early age of first marriage or first sexual intercourse; 5) many sex partners; 6) premarital sex; 7) extramarital sex; 8) illegitimacy; 9) poverty; 10) living in the city; 11) prostitution; and 12) syphilis.

Certainly, it is important to note that very few women with genital herpes actually develop cervical cancer and that many women who do have cancer of the cervix have never had herpes type-2.

Nonetheless, there is enough evidence now that there may be a connection between herpes and cancer that any woman with genital herpes should see her doctor regularly for an internal and external genital examination. The importance of the *Pap smear* in all women is well known. In women with genital herpes, this test should be done as close to every six to eight months as possible or, at the very least, once yearly. This will not only detect early cancerous changes but active herpes as well. If early malignant changes are found, treatment is highly effective and the *cure rate close to 100 percent*.

Vulval Cancer (External Genital Cancer)

Just as we have noticed an increase in cancer of the cervix, a similar type of localized cancer of the external genitalia in women is now being reported with increasing frequency. This increase, like cervical cancer, has been associated with herpes simplex type-2 infection, but the virus has yet to be proven as the causal agent of the disease. This local cancer or precancerous change of the external genitalia is called vulval CIS (carcinoma *in situ*). Nearly four out of every ten women who have this problem are younger than forty years of age and half of them have no knowledge of their illness at the time of diagnosis. Because vulval CIS is an *easily curable* illness which you may detect with self-examination, three short case reports are given below so that you may recognize the early signs of this genital problem. These cases were adapted from a study in which specific herpes simplex type-2 proteins were found in the malignant cells taken from women who had vulval CIS.[25]

Case 1: Patient number one had three recurrences of genital herpes during the six months before she developed growths on her external genitalia. Examination revealed raised pigmented bumps on the skin between the vagina and rectum, as well as on the genital lips on either side of the vaginal opening. A biopsy was diagnosed as CIS.

Case 2: Patient number two experienced an attack of primary genital herpes from which type-2 was cultured. Six weeks later, several clearly defined, raised, flat bumps were found on the genital lips, immediately next to the vaginal opening. Biopsy confirmed a diagnosis of CIS. One month later, a biopsy was taken from her cervix and revealed tissue changes which can be seen in the premalignant state.

Case 3: Patient number three had had a hysterectomy for cancer localized to her cervix six years before she developed problems with her external genitalia. The vulval changes were gray-white, slightly raised bumps on the inner side of the genital lips next to the vaginal opening. There were also pigmented lesions spreading back toward the rectum. A biopsy was diagnostic of vulval CIS.

The importance of the above descriptions is not only to teach you what you should look for in self-examinations but also to let you know that some changes which may seem to be malignant are not—and others may be *associated with changes in your cervix* which do need treatment. In addition, we know that these cell changes may occur within just a few weeks of herpes type-2 infection or many years later. In the study just described, one seventy-nine-year-old woman developed these changes many years after she had ceased sexual activity. Herpes type-2 specific proteins were found in her tumor cells as well. We should remember, however, that not all sores or bumps on your genitalia are either herpes or local cancer and *most are due to perfectly benign problems* which are easily treated; for example, genital warts. As in cancer of the cervix, the final proof that herpes infection causes malignant change has yet to be established. Nonetheless, any woman with a suspicious sore or bump on her genitalia should have a gynecologic examination, as *treatment of these lesions early on is simple and curative.*

11. NEURALGIC PAIN AND HERPES SIMPLEX VIRUS

Neuralgic pain is pain radiating down a leg, an arm, or across the face and is most commonly due to compression or irritation of a nerve root by a slipped disk or an arthritic bony spur. When we think of herpetic neuralgia, we most commonly think of herpes zoster and this is discussed more completely in that section. Herpes simplex virus, however, may also cause radiating neuralgic pain and should be considered as a possible cause of neuralgia in any patient with known herpetic infection.

The following cases describe two married couples in which both husband and wife had leg neuralgia associated with recurrent attacks of genital herpes simplex.[20]

Case 1: Husband number one developed episodes of sharp shooting pain radiating down both legs. These attacks of pain began three to four days before the appearance of itching and redness at the base of his penis. Blisters then appeared on the shaft of his penis and as they healed over the course of three days, the pain in his legs resolved. Over a three-year period, he had three to six recurrences of attacks characterized by leg pain followed a few days later by genital herpes. Herpes simplex type-2 was cultured from the blisters.

Case 2: The thirty-four-year-old wife of patient number one noted the onset of her leg pain approximately one year after her husband had noted his. She described the radiating leg pain as dull and nonthrobbing but made worse by walking. Her first attack of herpes ulcers occurred on the external genitalia and was not associated with leg pain. One month later, however, she had the onset of neuralgia and noted that with each recurrent attack the pain was followed by small blisters on her genitalia which healed over a seven-to-ten-day period. Herpes virus type-2 was cultured from her cervix during one of her neuralgic attacks.

Case 3: Husband number two had recurring neuralgic pain which radiated from the base of his spine along the outside of his leg to his foot. Two days after the onset of each attack of pain, small blisters would break out at the base of his spine and were associated with swollen glands in his groin. Herpes simplex type-2 was cultured from the blisters.

Case 4: Several months later, the thirty-four-year-old wife of husband number two noted the onset of the first of multiple attacks of pain in her pelvis radiating down the outside of both legs. At times the pain was shooting in nature and at other times it was dull and aching. A few days after each episode of pain began, she noticed the development of blisters on her external genitals. Virus cultures were negative, but her blood antibody levels to herpes virus were extremely high and compatible with recurrent herpetic infection.

All neurological and X-ray exams of these four patients were normal both during periods of neuralgic pain and in between recurrent episodes.

Although the exact incidence is not known, the pain of neuralgia as noted above is not uncommonly associated with herpes simplex. The four cases described above are somewhat more marked than usual but clearly show an association between leg pain and genital herpes infections. In addition, there have been reports of facial neuralgia similar to tic douloureux associated with recurring cold sores on the lips (type-1). Similarly, herpes infections of the fingers (whitlows) may be associated with neuralgia of the arm. In any case of neuralgia, then, herpes simplex—either type-1 or type-2—should be considered as a possible cause during the course of medical evaluation.

12. MOUTH AND SKIN INFECTIONS

Of all herpes infections in the country, disease around the mouth and skin are by far the most common. Nearly one hundred and eighty million people carry the virus somewhere in their bodies. About one hundred million of them develop overt attacks of herpes, know commonly as cold sores or fever blisters, at least once yearly. These recurrences, while annoying, are *harmless to the basically healthy person,* last only a few days, and heal without scarring. But while cold sores are essentially harmless to you when you have them, *they can spread the virus to someone else.* Refraining from kissing or other intimate contact and using your own towels, facecloths, and drinking glass is highly advisable. The cause of *mouth and skin infection* has, in the past, almost always been *type-1 herpes* virus, which *in these locations is non-venereal.* Increasingly, we see type-2 in adults, as there is a greater incidence of oral-genital contact during sexual activity. This is still infrequent but would be considered venereal because of the mode of spread. Type-2 contracted by a newborn during birth would *not be considered a venereal illness, however, as sexual activity was not involved. In fact, no herpes illness is venereal unless infection was by sexual activity.*

First Infection in the Mouth

Herpes of the mouth and face usually infects children under the age of five years. Fortunately, about 95 percent of these children experience no signs of illness or rash when this first infection comes. It is totally silent. The first time you discover that your child has oral or skin herpes is almost always when the first, or third, or fifth, recurrence occurs in the form of a small ulcer at the corner of the mouth or edge of the nostrils.

Very few children, then, develop noticeable disease, but when it is noticeable, it may be very severe and frightening, both to children and their parents. As bad as it may look, however, basically healthy children recover without any problem. Typically, a child will catch the virus from a friend or family member who has a cold sore. About two to ten days after being exposed to the virus, the child may develop a high fever, stop eating, and become very fretful. The mouth becomes sore and the gums, the inside of the mouth, and the lips turn very red and swollen. Many blisters appear in the same area and break down to raw red ulcers after a day or two. There is usually swelling of the glands in the neck and other parts of the body may become infected. An adult who has not already been infected with herpes may develop similar disease and be even sicker than a child. Fortunately, even without treatment, the fever and swelling disappear, the sores heal over without leaving any scars, and everything returns to normal after a week to ten days.

The following case report is that of a young man who developed this disease somewhat later in life and in association with primary infection of his fingers. It is similar to the oral illness seen in the few children who become sick when they first encounter herpes virus.[31]

This eighteen-year-old white man was referred to a dental clinic for evaluation of sores in his mouth. Examination revealed many ulcers scattered throughout his mouth and involving the gums and the roof of his mouth near his front teeth. It was also found at this time that he had ulcers on the nail beds of his right thumb and left little finger. These sores had started at the same time as those in his mouth and had been present for four days. Further questioning revealed that he had a habit of placing this thumb and finger in his mouth occasionally. His illness, which included a temperature of 101° F, indicated that he had a primary herpes infection, probably type-1, of his mouth and fingers.

No specific treatment was given, other than medication to assist symptomatically, such as aspirin and mouthwash. Just eleven days after the onset of his infection, his mouth had returned to its previous normal condition, but the sores on his fingers persisted. He now had blood-filled blisters on his little finger. Without specific therapy, however, his hand continued to improve and, by seven weeks after the onset of infection, had entirely returned to normal.

This case is unusual, not simply because of the age of the patient but because the sores on his fingers are probably due to herpes type-1. As I have indicated in the section discussing herpes of the fingers (see "Venereal Herpes Outside the Genital Area"), blisters involving the nail beds and sides of the fingers are often due to type-2 and indicate that you or someone you know may have genital herpes as well. As you have noted, however, in the section on infections of the fingers, there are obvious and very important *exceptions to this rule.*

Recurrent Herpes of the Mouth

During the first attack, whether it was noticeable or not, viruses have climbed through the nerves to the base of the brain and a portion of them go to sleep (become latent) in the deep nerve ganglion cells that run to the mouth and skin around it. Several months or years later, the virus may awaken again, usually because of fever or some other form of stress. It travels back down the nerves and reappears inside your mouth, nose or around your lips to produce the familiar blistering cold sores. Frequently, you will have some warning that the attack is about to begin. This may be numbness or a tingling sensation in the area. The blisters come in a few hours, break into red ulcers, crust over and heal without scarring all in a matter of a few days. Unlike a noticeable first attack you will have no fever or swelling of the neck glands unless you have some other infection such as the flu at the same time. You will also not have the same pain and discomfort in your mouth that a full blown first attack causes.

Herpes of the Skin—First Infection

The virus can affect the skin anywhere on your body. As mentioned, we generally feel that infections above the waist are most often caused by type-1 herpes and those below the waist or on the fingers by type-2. A first infection of the skin is usually very mild or not noticeable but on occasion may cause severe, widespread blistering and ulceration associated with fever, muscle aching, and swelling of local glands under your arms, in your groin, or your neck. The first attack lasts between ten to fourteen days and then heals completely without scarring.

Recurrent Herpes of the Skin

As in first mouth or genital infections, the virus travels quickly from the skin to your deep nerve ganglion centers, where it goes to sleep (becomes latent). Months or years later, various excitatory or stressful activities on your part may awaken the virus. It will travel back down the same nerves to produce another but much milder attack than the first one (if your first attack happened to have been a notable one).

In all cases, whether a first or a recurrent attack, the ulcers may be contagious to other people until the crusts are falling off. In recurrent attacks, this is on or before the fourth day after the start of the disease.

Diagnosis

As in genital herpes, the diagnosis is usually made by your doctor, based on what your mouth and skin look like. Occasionally, *other viruses such as herpangina may cause a similar mouth dis-*

ease. It is important to tell them apart, as herpangina does not come back again in recurrent attacks as herpes does and is, in fact, caused by the unrelated Group A coxsackievirus. Some bacterial infections of the skin may also look a bit like herpes. If there is a question, your doctor may gently take a smear from your infected area and look at it under the microscope to check for evidence of herpes. A blood test can also be useful. It will be sent to the State Virology Laboratory to check for antibodies against several different kinds of viruses. In large medical centers, there are often virus culture laboratories. Culturing the virus allows your doctor to determine if you have type-1 or type-2 herpes around your mouth or skin.

Treatment—General Measures

In a severe first attack of either the mouth or skin, general supportive therapy will do much to make you or your child feel better until the illness goes away on its own. This includes taking aspirin, aspirin-containing medications, or any drug you usually use to lower fever, to reduce muscle aching, and to relieve general feelings of being unwell. If pain is unusually severe, your doctor may give you stronger drugs (such as codeine) for a few days to help you through. Aspirin or other antifever drugs may be used with this medication to keep the fever down.

For either a first infection or discomforting recurrent infection, saltwater mouthwashes (one teaspoon table salt per quart of cool water) will help cleanse the lesions and reduce swelling. If you do have sores in the mouth, it is best not to eat solid foods for a few days, as this will just traumatize the ulcers more. Milk, custards, gelatin, and soups are the best forms of nourishment to take during this period. It is important to keep up adequate intake of fluids.

For skin ulcers, cool tap water compresses for five minutes twice daily, using a wet facecloth or small towel, followed by gentle but thorough drying, will help to keep the ulcers clean and provide comfort. Remember, *keep these cloths separate* from those used by other people, as they are contagious. Launder them frequently with detergent. Your doctor may also provide further comfort for you in the form of numbing anesthetic ointments or liquids (such as lidocaine) or anti-inflammation ointments from the cortisone group of drugs. Use of *cortisone* in infectious disease has been questioned by some physicians. Although there is evidence that it does decrease cell damage, it may spread the disease further. Whether your own doctor uses it depends on his judgment as to what will be best and safest for you. *Drying agents,* such as 5 percent salt or 4 percent boric acid ointment are available in drugstores, and are generally safe when used four times daily for five days. Many doctors, however, feel that just keeping the area *clean and dry* is *preferable to keeping it moist under an ointment.*

Antiviral Drugs

In the many studies which are done in an attempt to find treatment for herpes infection of cold sores around the nose and mouth, we have learned that the body mounts its natural defense mechanisms against the recurrent infection within twenty-four hours of the onset of your illness. Nonetheless, during the few days when you have a cold sore, you are infectious and capable of spreading herpes type-1, either to the facial region of someone who has not previously been infected or to the genital area during lovemaking. It is important, therefore, to develop medication which can shorten the period of time during which you are capable of spreading this virus to those who are close to you.

Antiviral drugs available to your doctor (idoxuridine, vidarabine, trifluridine) are of no use on the skin or mouth. Others more recently reported (Ara-AMP, phosphonoacetic or phosphonoformic acid, PAA or PFA) are not generally available and, after much testing, have not been shown to be effective and safe. The following study is more encouraging with reference to our bodies' own ability to handle the situation, with or without antiviral drugs.[45]

Ninety-three patients were entered into this study. They had been studied previously in an antiviral trial in which they had been given either Ara-AMP or acyclovir. This earlier study had been a failure because no significant difference could be found between the drug-treated patients and those who had received placebos (drugless ointment). The present study revealed that the pain, size of the cold sores, and the number of viruses present in the ulcers were greatest in the patients who were examined within the first eight hours of the onset of their symptoms. When patients were seen after eight hours or later, they had already begun to improve with respect to all three of these factors. The conclusion reached from this study was that, in order to treat cold sores effectively and protect both you and your companion from spread of infection, treatment must be started within eight hours. As we know from other studies using drugs such as acyclovir, this early therapy will rapidly reduce the numbers of virus present in the sores at least in first infections and therefore reduce the period during which you are infectious and capable of spreading the disease.

Dietary Therapy

Dietary therapy in the form of bioflavinoids (*Vitamin P*) and, more particularly, *L-lysine* tablets (a protein building block) have received considerable publicity as common health foods which prevent recurrent attacks of herpes and shorten those which occur. L-lysine is felt to interfere with the creation of new herpes virus particles and is commonly sold in health food stores. It is generally taken in a total dose of 1,000 milligrams per day, usually as a 312-milligram tablet three times daily or one 500-milligram tablet two times daily. All evidence is not yet in on this pill, but it appears to be harmless in the dose prescribed. Many patients feel very strongly that they can prevent an attack if they take the pills at the first tingle or warning sign. Others feel that those attacks they do have are much milder if they take L-lysine. The results of scientific studies do not agree as to whether the drug really works or whether people just think they are better because they feel they are doing something about their herpes. The current opinion by a number of experts is that there may be a few people for whom the tablets do have some effect, but this is probably *more psychological than biological*. Doctors do not yet know how to predict which patients, if any, may or may not benefit from taking L-lysine. Further studies are under way.

Solvents

Other forms of treatment which you may have heard of are now felt to be not very effective or dangerous. If used at all, they must be given only by a doctor or directly under his or her supervision. Liquids, such as alcohol, ether, or chloroform, dissolve the fat in the virus wall, making them noninfectious, but probably do not speed healing. However, the dangers of ether, in terms of its explosiveness and highly poisonous nature if breathed in excessively, have already been mentioned under genital herpes. Chloroform has been banned by the Food and Drug Administration for use in any new drugs or domestic products because there is now evidence that it may cause cancer in mice. This leaves only alcohol and there is very little proof that it has much good effect.

Dye-Light Therapy (Photodynamic Inactivation)

This therapy was widely publicized recently as an effective treatment for herpes of the skin, lips, or genitalia. It had been found that painting the sores with certain dyes resulted in the dyes binding with the genetic material of the viruses. Exposure to ordinary fluorescent light then resulted in the virus material breaking up, thus being inactivated. While early work was very encouraging, studies have now shown that the effect on disease is minimal and does nothing to prevent another attack later. There is also some concern that the viruses themselves could possibly be changed to produce local malignant disease, although this has not yet been proven.

Vaccines

The use of currently available vaccines or drugs which might increase your body's ability to fight herpes virus with white cells and antibodies has also fallen by the wayside as forms of therapy. Vaccines (such as BCG or Lupidon) and drugs (such as levamisole) fail to shorten a current attack or prevent another one. Better vaccines are now being developed (see "Hope for the Future").

In summary, the most effective therapy for herpes of the mouth or skin is aspirin or aspirinlike drugs for fever, careful daily cleansing and drying, and possibly the application of nonirritating drying solutions or ointments.

13. HERPES AND INFECTIONS OF THE BRAIN

The most common forms of brain infections are meningitis (infection of the membranes wrapped around the brain and spinal cord) and encephalitis (infection of the brain substance itself). When we think of meningitis, we usually think of a highly lethal or damaging disease which, in fact, is caused most commonly by bacteria, not viruses. If caught early, antibiotic treatment is highly effective. On rare occasions, however, meningitis may be caused by herpes simplex virus. Unlike the more common bacterial meningitis, herpes infections of the membranes around the brain and spinal cord are a fairly benign illness.

Encephalitis is an infection or inflammation of the brain substance itself. It may be highly localized or spread diffusely throughout the tissues. Most commonly, this illness is caused by viruses, such as "horse" (equine) encephalitis, but herpes is high on the list as the agent responsible for the majority of these cases. Fortunately, encephalitis itself is also rare. Even though herpes causes many such infections, then, it is still a very uncommon illness but very serious when it occurs. Early treatment is paramount and available.

It is important to know the early signs and symptoms of both meningitis and encephalitis, so that you will get to your doctor or to a hospital emergency service immediately if you detect them. It may or may not be herpes, but either illness needs treatment, regardless of its cause.

Meningitis

Genital herpes, type-2, is most commonly assciated with meningitis and is probably a result of virus spread from the genitalia to the deep nerve ganglia along the spinal cord and then to the membranes themselves. Occasionally, type-1 virus may spread from the mouth to the fifth nerve ganglia at the base of the brain, then to the membranes, causing similar disease. The infection itself occurs in both sexes of all ages and, when it does occur, is often associated with recurrent genital or mouth herpes. Fortunately, herpes meningitis is a rather harmless—although alarming —disease. There is usually severe headache, stiff neck, fever, and some confusion of thought. Unlike herpes encephalitis, there is no loss of consciousness or convulsion.

Diagnosis is made by neurological examination, spinal tap, and occasionally by special X rays.

There is no treatment, other than fluids, aspirinlike drugs, and general support. Patients usually recover completely within a month, but occasionally there may be recurrent attacks. One patient was known to have had seventeen cases of genital herpes associated with meningitis during a fourteen-year period.

While meningitis is, in general, considered an extremely dangerous illness when bacteria are involved, then, in the case of herpes simplex it can be a distressing but essentially harmless infection of the membranes which surround the brain. The following cases will give you some idea of the nature of this illness.[41]

The patients ranged in age from sixteen to twenty-six years of age, six women and one man. Of the seven, six had a benign herpetic meningitis, with fever lasting only two to three days and rapidly clearing symptoms. The seventh patient had fever for a week and persistent headache, instability of his moods, difficulty speaking (dysphoria), and feelings of extreme exhaustion lasting ten months. All patients denied cold sores about the mouth, but two had noticed blisters in the genital region approximately one week before the onset of symptoms characterized by fever, headache, and a stiff neck. One patient developed a measleslike rash over the face and neck and two had sharp neuralgic pains in their legs for a few days before the onset of the meningitis.

Spinal fluid samples were consistent with a diagnosis of meningitis, but brain wave tests were normal in five and only temporarily abnormal in two patients.

Five to seven months after the first episode of meningitis, two patients developed recurrent benign episodes of the same illness.

When we compare the headache of meningitis with encephalitis, we can see that the former is a harmless illness indeed, while the latter is highly damaging, potentially fatal, but, fortunately, very rare (see also "Herpes in the Newborn Child" and "Herpes in Pregnant Women").

Encephalitis

Herpes infection is very uncommon but still is the most common cause of acute viral infection of the brain itself. We do not yet know the exact incidence. It is caused most commonly by *nonvenereal type-1 herpes* but occasionally by type-2 in association with genital infection. Untreated, the infection may be a severe, rapidly progressive, and potentially fatal disease. The virus causes destruction in various parts of the brain. At its onset, patients have flulike symptoms, such as fever, headache, and drowsiness. Virus blisters may then appear on the mouth, skin, or genital region. Soon comes the onset of stiff neck, delirium, inability to move certain muscles or limbs, convulsions, and, without treatment (and sometimes with), coma and death.

The doctor makes the diagnosis based on examination of the patient, spinal taps, electronic brain scans, special X rays, blood tests, and often a surgical brain biopsy.

Once the diagnosis is confirmed or even reasonably suspected, antiviral treatment with intravenous vidarabine or acyclovir* is begun. Drugs or surgery to take pressure off the swollen brain may also be used. *The earlier the therapy is begun, the better the chances for a good recovery.* There may, however, be some brain damage left, despite the best treatment available. Cases of herpes encephalitis in newborn infants and adults are described under "Pregnancy, Birth, and the Newborn Baby."

* Acyclovir is not yet FDA-approved for treatment of herpetic encephalitis.

14. HERPES AND OUR EYES—KERATITIS AND IRITIS

While herpes simplex is the most common cause of blindness due to infection in the entire North American continent, it is still infrequent with only one of every four hundred to six hundred people having an attack of herpes in the eye, and very few of these people ever go on to lose vision. Almost all infections are confined to one eye with the other eye never getting a herpes infection. In fact, only about one of twelve hundred people who already have herpes of one eye ever have the second eye involved. The most common cause of *ocular herpes is type 1* and is *nonvenereal*. Again, because of the many changes and variety in our sexual activities, we see rare but increasing numbers of type-2 infection around the mouth and in the eyes of adults. Newborn babies born of mothers with genital herpes are also at special risk of developing type-2 herpes infections in their eyes (see "Pregnancy, Birth, and the Newborn Baby"). Both types of herpes, 1 and 2, produce the same disease in the eyes and, fortunately, both types are equally susceptible to the antiviral treatment we have available. Diagnosis and therapy are carried out by your ophthalmologist.

First Infection

It is rare to have a first infection involving the eyes. When it does occur, it is almost always in young children and may be quite severe with fever, swelling of the lids, blistering and raw sores of the skin around the eyes, redness of the eyes themselves, and ulceration of the clear window at the front of the eye, the cornea. Even without treatment, first infections will generally heal completely within two to three weeks, but treatment greatly hastens the end of the disease. There is no residual scarring from the virus.

Recurrent Infected Eye Ulcers

A recurrent attack of infected ulceration of the eye is not necessarily preceded by a first attack in your eye. Most eye infections, in fact, occur in patients who had their first attack, noticeable or not, in the mouth. During the first attack in your mouth, the herpes virus travels through the nerves leading from your lips, gums, or skin of your face to the deep nerve ganglion centers at the base of your brain. The main nerve center involved is called the fifth nerve (trigeminal) ganglion. The fifth nerve sends fibers not only to the lower part of your face but to your eyes as well. Therefore, virus can get into your ganglion through the nerves from your mouth, sleep there in latency for weeks, months, or years, and then suddenly reawaken. Once awake and actively producing infectious viruses, this source of herpes may send some of the viruses out through the nerves which just happen to go to your eye. Your mouth or nose may or may not have another attack at that time. Once in your eye, the virus causes it to become sore, red, and watery. Vision blurs as ulcers develop on your cornea (keratitis) and deep, aching pain may indicate that the virus has also gotten into your iris, the blue or brown part of your eye (iritis). This causes inflammation deep inside your eye which, if allowed to go untreated, may lead to glaucoma (elevated eye pressure) or, rarely, cataract (cloudy lens) formation.

If you once have an attack of herpes in your eye, you stand about a 25 percent chance of a second attack there within five years. If that attack occurs, your chances of yet a third attack double again—to nearly 50 percent—in the next five years. With each attack, the chances of another seem to increase. Fortunately, as noted above, herpes almost never involves both eyes. Those very few patients who do have both eyes infected usually started having attacks when they were children. After a series of recurrences over one or two years, it is not unusual for the infections to stop coming as suddenly as they started. The reason for this spontaneous "cure" is not known.

Loss of Vision

The ulcers themselves rarely cause enough scarring to cause great loss of vision. Herpes impairs an eye by a different mechanism. Each time some virus travels down to your cornea or inside your eye to the iris, it causes changes in your own eye tissues. These changes make the infected cells take on some characteristics that your body recognizes as a herpes virus. It sees your own corneal and iris tissues as foreign, invading germs and tries to attack and reject them, much as it would try to reject a foreign kidney transplant. It is as if you had become allergic to your own eye. When your body rejects tissue, it attacks it by sending white blood cells and antibodies specially programmed against the tissue. In the case of herpes in your eye, the cells and antibodies attack the tissues which have been changed to seem like herpes virus. The result is inflammation—a red and sometimes painful eye. If no treatment is given and the attack continues, more and more eye tissue becomes damaged and scarred. Your cornea is no longer a clear window to the inside of your eye but a swollen, hazy, scarred tissue that prevents your eye from seeing clearly. As scarring worsens with each allergic attack, vision through the corneal window may be lost altogether and your eye becomes blind.

In some cases, your cornea may cloud from allergic attack and its surface break down in ulcers which do not heal because your eye is so damaged by viral and inflammatory changes. In this situation, there is danger that the ulcers will move deeper through the cornea.

If the iris is persistently attacked and not treated, it may scar to the inside of the eye, causing glaucoma. This persistently high pressure in your eye can cause vision loss by slowly damaging the visual nerve. Cataract may also develop and cause loss of vision because your eye's lens is so cloudy.

Diagnosis

Like most other forms of herpes, ocular infection is almost always diagnosed by what your eye looks like when your ophthalmologist examines it. The infected ulcers are usually very easy to recognize. The scarring from inflammatory allergic reaction is also often quite easily diagnosed, but, on occasion, other eye diseases may look very much like herpes. In these cases, it is helpful to the doctor if you let him or her know whether you have had a known attack of herpes in your eye before or if you have some cold sores on your face at the time of your eye problem. Cold sores mean that the virus is active in the fifth nerve ganglion that sends fibers both to your face and eye.

Diagnostic tests which may be done, if necessary, include taking scrapings (after an anesthetic eye drop is given) for study under a microscope, taking virus cultures for growth in a laboratory, or taking blood samples to test for antiherpes antibody levels.

Treatment with Antiviral and Antiallergy Drugs

Until the recent FDA approval of acyclovir for certain forms of genital and skin herpes, the brain and the eye were the only places in the body where we truly had specific antiviral drugs which worked and were commercially available. For treating infected eye ulcers there are now three drugs sold in your local drugstores. IDU (Stoxil™, Herplex™, Dendrid™) comes as an ointment used five times daily or as an eye drop used every hour by day and every two hours at night—usually for two to three weeks. Vidarabine (Vira-A™) is an ointment used five times daily and trifluridine (Viroptic™) is a drop used nine times daily for two to three weeks. All three drugs are very effective in eliminating virus from your eye. Acyclovir is also an excellent antiviral in the eye but currently awaits FDA review for that use. If you become allergic or sensitive to one drug, your eye doctor can switch you to another for future treatment. Unfortunately, although the drugs almost always heal in the ulcers, they act only on the surface of the eye and can do nothing to get rid of the deep virus stored in the deep nerve ganglia. This means that the drugs are good once an attack starts but do nothing to prevent another attack coming down from the ganglia later.

If you have the allergic form of herpes in your eye, your doctor may have to use cortisone-type eye medications or pills to quiet the inflammation and to prevent scarring or growth of abnormal blood vessels. If cortisone is being used in your eye, it decreases the eye's ability to fight infection. Your doctor will often use antiviral and antibacterial drugs along with it to protect the eye, not just against infectious herpes but against bacterial germ invasion as well. In addition, you will be checked from time to time for glaucoma (which, if present, will be treated with eye drops or pills) or cataracts. Cortisone can cause either of these. Often it is impossible to tell whether these complications are from the herpes disease, from the treatment, or from both. Your doctor will not keep you on cortisone any longer than is necessary to control the allergic attack on your eye, although a few patients must stay on a daily or weekly eye drop for years. In many cases, if this attack is not controlled with cortisonelike drugs, the eye will lose vision from the disease anyway. As with any illness, *it is often necessary to risk some complications of treatment in order to save your sight.*

Therapeutic Soft Contact Lenses

Occasionally, even though the antiviral drugs have cleared all virus from the eye, the ulcers do not heal in because of mechanical damage to the tissue. If an ulcer stays open too long, it may cause the eye to rupture. Special thin, clear, soft contact lenses are used to treat sterile ulcers. The lens is put in by your doctor and left in day and night for weeks or months. It protects the front of your eye from the rubbing action of your lid when you blink, thus allowing your eye's surface to heal under the lens.

Corneal Transplants

Occasionally, despite the best of care, the body's attacks on the cornea are too much and the front of the eye scars over to cause blindness. In such cases, your doctor may recommend a corneal transplant by an eye surgeon specialized in that field. This means replacing your scarred cornea with a new clear one. If you happen to have a bad cataract, your eye surgeon may remove it at the same time your transplant is done. Depending on how badly your eye is damaged, your chances of regaining vision range from 90 percent success down to about 50 percent success. If your new transplant does fail and cloud again, however, it may be replaced by yet another clear cornea. Corneal transplants are not a once-only opportunity and may be repeated if necessary.

Other Forms of Treatment

1) *Chemical wiping.* In the days before antiviral drugs were developed, treatment involved rubbing the ulcer with a cotton-tipped stick soaked in a chemical such as iodine or ether. It was highly effective therapy but sometimes caused problems with healing because of the toxic effects of the chemicals. Today, eye physicians often still wipe off the ulcers (and much virus) with a cotton-tip, but many no longer use the chemicals. They then start antiviral treatment.

2) *Interferon.* This is a natural protein-sugar substance produced by your body cells in reaction to attack by viruses or certain chemicals. It blocks development of new viruses by stimulating yet another body chemical that interferes with important enzymes necessary for virus growth. Interferon eye drops have been used to treat human ulcers with only short-term success. Interferon is now being studied for use as a daily eye drop used to prevent eye infections and as treatment for an ulcer once it has developed.

3) *Dye-light therapy (Photodynamic Inactivation).* This is discussed more extensively under "Mouth and Skin Infections." It was used with some success in the eye, but several patients had toxic inflammatory reactions. It is no longer used for herpes of the eye.

4) *L-lysine* is also discussed under "Mouth and Skin Infections." There are no studies in the eye showing that L-lysine tablets work for herpes infections. If it is true that certain people in the country do benefit from L-lysine therapy for herpes of the skin or genitalia—and this is doubtful at best—one may hope that certain people with eye infections would benefit from the L-lysine. Unfortunately, we don't know how to predict who, if anyone, will benefit and who will not. The effect is more likely psychological than truly medical. My own studies in this area have shown no therapeutic effect.

5) *Ara-AMP*. This is an antiviral drug related to the commercially available vidarabine (Ara-A). While initial studies showed that this drug was very effective in treating herpes ulcers of the eye, its irritating toxic side effects made it unsuitable for general use.

While about 90 percent of ocular herpes infections heal in quickly and without complications, the following two case reports from my own practice are presented as examples of the progression of successes and problems that doctors may rarely encounter in managing difficult herpes infections of the eye. It does not seem to matter whether the virus is type-1 or type-2. Each appears to cause the same disease and responds similarly to therapy.

Case Reports[34]

Case 1: This fifty-year-old man had been successfully treated for recurring herpes ulcers of both eyes since he was ten years of age. Ultimately, however, his corneas began to scar and he became legally blind in both eyes. To make matters worse, he had become violently allergic to IDU, the only antiviral agent available at that time. This meant that he could not have a corneal transplant because there was no antiviral agent which could be used during the postoperative period while cortisone drugs were in use.

By good fortune, vidarabine was being studied as a possible new antiviral drug for use in the eye. The patient was put on a regimen of cortisone eye drops to cause the abnormal blood vessels in the cornea to shrink and vidarabine ointment was used to prevent any infectious ulcers from developing. The trial was a success and it was decided to proceed with surgery.

One month later, he underwent an uncomplicated corneal transplant on his right eye. He successfully tolerated his postoperative cortisone and vidarabine. Six months after his surgery, he had excellent 20/20 vision in the transplanted eye and was taking no medication for his eye. The transplant has remained clear for the ten years since it was first put in.

Case 2: This twenty-six-year-old man developed a herpes ulcer in his left eye. It healed in rapidly with IDU eye drops. Unfortunately, he suffered a reactivation of herpes infection in that eye just a few months later. This time the IDU did not heal the ulcer and it was felt that the virus had become resistant to it. He was, therefore, placed on vidarabine ointment. Within a week, the ulcer was almost entirely healed, except for a small central area. Virus cultures were taken and were negative, indicating that the persistent ulcer was no longer due to the presence of virus but to a mechanical problem in healing due to excessive tissue damage.

Despite the use of a therapeutic soft contact lens which the patient wore continuously day and night, the ulcer persisted. Three months later, enzymes released by the sick tissue around the ulcer caused the eye to perforate. Because the eye was so soft and leaking fluid, it was felt that surgery would be dangerous. Instead the perforation site was sealed with a surgical form of Super Glue™. The leak stopped; the eye firmed up and became less inflamed.

Six months later, he underwent an uncomplicated corneal transplant. While his transplant remained very clear during the postoperative period, however, his vision was poor because an early cataract had formed prior to the perforation and worsened after it.

One year after the transplant, he could see almost nothing from his eye because the cataract had ripened. He therefore underwent a successful cataract operation with resulting vision wearing a contact lens being a good 20/40.

In the two years since his last operation, he has had no recurrence of herpes and continues to do well.

15. HERPES OF THE DIGESTIVE TRACT

Although the exact incidence is not known, herpes may occasionally involve the digestive tube (esophagus) leading from your mouth to your stomach. Most patients who have this have years of heartburn (deep central chest pain) "acid indigestion," or severe difficulty and pain on swallowing but very rarely develop bleeding problems. A most important part of the diagnosis includes making sure that you don't have one of the other more common causes of these symptoms, such as a stomach or duodenal ulcer, hiatus hernia, gall bladder or heart disease, chronic inflammation of the stomach, or abnormal enlargement of the blood vessels associated with liver problems.

If the problem warrants it, your doctor may need to look down your digestive tube. If you have herpes, he or she will see many typical small viral ulcers inside the tube. The most common cause is type-1 herpes and is *nonvenereal,* but there is no reason why swallowing type-2 herpes couldn't cause it. Unless there is bleeding, the disease is uncomfortable with each recurrent attack but *not dangerous.* Treatment includes common antacids and occasionally drinking a numbing anesthetic drug (viscous lidocaine) if there is much pain. The disease goes away by itself in a few days.

The following are case reports describing herpes infection of the upper intestinal tract. As you can see, all patients have severe pain on swallowing but even bleeding may rarely be the first sign of this infection.[33]

> This twenty-nine-year-old male physician had been in good health until he developed what appeared to be an upper respiratory tract infection, with sore throat, fever, and muscle aches. Ten days later, he developed severe pain on swallowing which was not relieved by liquid antacids. He then noticed the onset of severe pain deep in the center of his chest but had no nausea, vomiting, or heartburn. He did note, however, that his newlywed wife had had a recurrence of fever blisters on her mouth approximately three weeks before the onset of his own illness.
>
> X-ray studies of the upper intestinal tract were normal, but a direct examination of his esophagus (digestive tube) revealed that he had many superficial ulcers scattered throughout his esophagus and that there was diffuse bleeding throughout this region. Cultures taken from this area grew out herpes simplex type-1 virus. Additional blood tests showed that the patient's blood immune defense system was entirely normal.

He was treated symptomatically with antacids, viscous lidocaine (the liquid anesthetic that is swallowed) and tranquilizers. Within three days, he felt remarkably better. On the tenth day, he suddenly became anemic and was found to have blood in his bowel movement, probably the result of bleeding from the herpes ulcers. He was treated with iron pills and recovered without difficulty.

The next case presented in a much more dramatic fashion, in that this woman did not seek medical advice when her symptoms began but only when she suffered an episode of bleeding.[16]

This sixty-eight-year-old white woman had had mild intermittent burning deep in her chest typical of heartburn for several years. This heartburn was not affected by eating but became worse if she lay down after she had eaten. It was relieved by antacids. She was not nauseated and she had no difficulty swallowing or pain on swallowing.

On the day she came to the hospital, it was because she had begun to vomit blood and had passed a black bowel movement. She was pale, her pulse was rapid, and she was in moderate distress. There were no cold sores or ulcers found around her mouth. Her black bowel movement was positive for blood.

Examination of her upper digestive tract with the viewing tube revealed multiple ulcerations covered with white exudates. There was active bleeding in the lower two thirds of the esophagus but no abnormality below this. Virus cultures taken from this region grew out herpes simplex virus type-1.

Treatment included transfusion of whole blood, hourly antacids, and an antacid pill every six hours. Her bleeding stopped and she felt remarkably better. Ten days later, a repeat examination of the esophagus revealed healing of the ulcers.

The following cases demonstrate that herpes infections of the upper digestive tract may be found in young and very healthy patients. It may be a source of pain without any evidence of bleeding.[43]

Case 1: This twenty-year-old man complained of severe pain on swallowing. Examination of the upper digestive tract with the viewing tube revealed many punched-out ulcerations. Biopsy of this area showed typical herpes simplex inclusion bodies in the cells. Three days later, this man developed many herpes lesions on his hands and feet and virus cultures grew out herpes simplex type-1. Blood tests indicated that he had an entirely healthy blood immune defense system. He recovered totally from his illness within thirteen days.

Case 2: This otherwise healthy seventeen-year-old woman awoke suddenly with pain deep in her central chest area. She then developed pain when swallowing either solid or liquid food, although there was no difficulty in passage of the food through to her stomach. Two days later, she developed flulike symptoms which lasted for two days. When examined, X-ray tests were normal, but direct viewing of her upper digestive tract revealed small punched-out ulcers. Three days later, she developed herpes ulcers on her lips. Twelve days after the onset of her pain on swallowing, she was completely normal and repeat viewing of the esophagus was also normal.

Herpes infection of the upper digestive tract can also be seen in older patients, particularly those with some other form of debilitating disease. The following three cases are of interest because one is in an older women who had an associated duodenal ulcer (peptic ulcer) in her middle intestinal tract, the second case because the patient was on therapy with a potent antiviral drug at the time he developed his herpetic illness, and the third case because antiviral treatment was successfully used.[39]

Case 1: This seventy-two-year-old woman had symptoms of recurring pain in her midabdominal area just below the chest cage for eight months. This was associated with nausea, vomiting, poor appetite, and a thirty-pound weight loss. She also complained of heartburn and intermittent problems of swallowing solid food but no pain on swallowing. Special X-ray studies revealed marked scarring of the small intestinal area just beyond the stomach. This was due to acute and chronic peptic ulcer disease. A direct viewing of the upper digestive tract, however, also revealed many oval ulcerations covered in exudate. Biopsies from these areas showed changes typical of herpes simplex infection. A repeat direct viewing several days after she had had surgery for her peptic ulcer revealed that her herpetic disease had completely healed.

Case 2: This fifty-one-year-old man had acute leukemia and was being treated with cytosine-arabinoside, a somewhat toxic drug used both for therapy of leukemia and occasionally for herpes simplex infection. Eight days after the start of treatment, he developed a fever and complained of pain on swallowing. He was treated with various antibiotics, but because he became worse he underwent direct viewing of the upper intestinal tract with the viewing tube. This test revealed that he had many ulcers and plaques which were quite fragile and bled easily. Biopsy taken from this area showed changes typical of herpes simplex infection. The patient had no evidence of herpes infection in or about his mouth. A repeat of the direct viewing test in the upper digestive tract twenty days later showed marked improvement in the herpetic disease.

Case 3: This thirty-seven-year-old man noted pain and difficulty on swallowing while undergoing a four-week course of X-ray therapy for cancer of the lung. He had not suffered any heartburn, nausea, vomiting, or acid regurgitation. On examination, he had no signs of herpes infection around his mouth, but his stool was positive for blood. X-ray studies showed changes consistent with herpes infection of the upper intestinal tract. This was confirmed by direct viewing of the esophagus. Biopsy showed cell changes characteristic of herpes simplex infection.

This patient was treated with intravenous acyclovir with rapid improvement in his symptoms.

In addition to being a cause of ulceration in the upper digestive tract, herpes simplex has been associated with the occurrence of peptic (duodenal) ulcers in the intestinal tract just beyond the stomach. The evidence for this is rather circumstantial and includes such factors as: 1) peptic ulcers and herpes infection are both most common in the spring and fall; 2) both illnesses are more common in people with blood type O; 3) patients with peptic ulcers have higher levels of herpes type-1 antibodies than patients with herpetic antibodies but no ulcers; and 4) the levels of herpes type-1 antibodies in ulcer patients rises in a manner similar to those seen in some patients with recurring cold sores of their lips.[5]

16. ATHLETICS AND HERPES

Just as certain occupations such as dentistry are associated with a higher than normal incidence of herpes infection of the fingers, certain athletic activities may be associated with high incidence of *nonvenereal* herpes infection elsewhere in the body. Most prominent among these is herpes simplex infection among wrestlers. Because of the nature of its spread, it tends to occur in epidemic form. In one epidemic at a prominent New England college in 1965, seven of nineteen wrestlers developed herpes infections of the right side of the face, forearms, swollen glands in the neck, and varying degrees of conjunctivitis. Involvement of the right side of the head and face is probably the result of a wrestling maneuver known as "locking-up" or "closed position standing." A right-handed wrestler places his hand on his opponent's neck and pulls him forward, bringing the right side of his head into direct contact with that of his opponent. In an attempt to intimidate and unbalance their opponents, wrestlers then engage their scalps, hair, or beard in a rough, grinding fashion. Any herpes virus present at this time would easily be inoculated into the skin and spread across the face and to the forearms as they grasp their opponents' necks.

The following is just one of six cases reported after an epidemic of herpes among the wrestling team at a large Southern university.[49]

A twenty-year-old male wrestler developed blisters on his right cheek. Within a week, almost the entire cheek was involved, as well as the skin behind the right ear, the external area of both ears, and part of the left cheek. There were swollen glands and fever. Five days later, crusting was present and the sores were healing by themselves.

Two days after wrestling with the above patient, a teammate, also age twenty, developed blisters on the right cheek, forehead, and portions of his neck. He did not feel ill, but the sores were quite painful. Crusting and healing began within two weeks. Cultures taken from these patients were positive for herpes simplex virus. It appears likely that the second teammate contracted his herpes while wrestling with the first. These infections were subsequently spread to four other members of the team.

Unfortunately, this team also wrestled with a group from a college in an adjacent state. Within ten days, herpes infections of the face broke out in three members of the out-of-state team. It seems apparent that, in addition to spreading the infection among themselves, the first team easily spread the herpes infection to members of another team through use of the locking-up maneuver.

While wrestling is the most obvious area in which herpes may be spread from athlete to athlete, other contact sports such as football, rugby, or soccer are not necessarily free of such complications.

Nonetheless, we should not avoid contact sports for fear of picking up herpes, as this is highly unlikely. If someone has obvious cold sores, however, it would be advisable for him or her to defer playing for a few days to protect others. Coaches and team doctors can make this decision.

17. ARTHRITIS AND HERPES

While the most common causes of arthritis (inflammation of the joints) are rheumatoid or degenerative, some forms may be infectious. The most well known of these is gonococcal (clap) infection of the joints, but the following case report indicates that herpes simplex is capable of producing a *nonvenereal acute arthritis* as well.[38]

> An eighteen-year-old college wrestler developed extensive crusting blisters on his forearms, neck, forehead, and scalp over a five-day period. He was admitted to the hospital when his right knee became extremely tender, hot, and swollen. The slightest movement caused him marked pain in the knee and the admitting diagnosis was herpes gladiatorum (see "Athletics and Herpes") with an associated arthritis.
>
> The patient had had herpes zoster when four years of age but denied ever having had cold sores or fever blisters. Other than the lesions just described, he had no evidence of herpes infection elsewhere in the body. Cultures of the skin grew out herpes simplex type-1. A needle was placed in the right knee and fluid withdrawn for examination and culture. This too grew out herpes simplex type-1.
>
> The young man was treated with topical antiviral IDU (idoxuridine), antibiotic pills, and bed rest. Over the ensuing five days, the skin lesions dried and cleared and the swelling in his knee subsided. Within two weeks, he was back to full activity with no difficulties from his previously arthritic knee. It was subsequently learned that two of his wrestling team-mates had also developed widespread herpes after having wrestled with the patient just before his hospitalization.

18. HERPES ZOSTER (SHINGLES)

Zoster and Chicken Pox

Herpes zoster virus and chicken pox virus are one and the same. *They never cause venereal disease.* The first time you catch this virus, you get chicken pox and are usually covered with sores which blister, crust over, and heal, with little or no scarring. But during your first attack, the chicken pox virus, like the herpes simplex virus, probably travels to the deep nerve ganglion centers responsible for feeling pain and touch. These are located along the spinal cord and at the base of the brain. There, like simplex virus, the chicken pox virus apparently goes to sleep in a state of latency. Months (or more often years) later, something in one of the ganglia wakes up the virus. But this time it causes disease very different from chicken pox.

We commonly think of chicken pox as a harmless though annoying infection of childhood. On rare occasions, however, it can produce a very severe illness, particularly when it strikes patients who are in their teens or older. The following case report describes just such an episode and the successful outcome, thanks to therapy with the new antiviral drug, acyclovir.[47]

This patient was a twenty-five-year-old woman who had never had chicken pox as a child. One day her son developed the usual form of chicken pox and his mother was, of course, exposed to this highly contagious illness as she cared for him. She was in excellent health for three weeks during his illness and then suddenly experienced severe pain deep in her chest and exhaustion. The symptoms continued unabated and she developed a fever and noticed blisters breaking out in her mouth and across her face. Within twenty-four hours, these blisters had spread over the trunk of her body and she began to have difficulty breathing. She began to cough and to have pain in her chest when she attempted to inhale. Two days later, she became nauseated, developed a severe headache, and became drowsy and delirious. She was admitted to the hospital for treatment with antiviral therapy.

When she was admitted, her chest X ray revealed an extensive widespread viral pneumonia and her electrocardiogram indicated inflammation of her heart. Tests of her spinal fluid were normal. She was treated immediately with intravenous acyclovir* for five days. Within twenty-four hours, she improved dramatically. She was able to breathe with ease and very few new blisters developed. Her headache resolved and temperature returned to normal. Three days into

* Acyclovir is not FDA-approved for therapy of herpes zoster pneumonia.

her treatment, her chest X ray was much improved and, after treatment for a secondary bacterial pneumonia with antibiotics, she continued on to a rapid recovery. On the sixth day after treatment, her chest X ray was entirely normal and the inflammation in her heart had disappeared. There was no evidence of any abnormal side effects from use of the acyclovir.

We can see from this patient's clinical course that chicken pox pneumonia in an adult is a very serious and life-threatening disease. Although we can not state with 100 percent certainty that she would not have recovered without acyclovir, her rapid improvement once treatment was started was very convincing and indicates that we do have therapy for such severe involvement with chicken pox virus.

Fortunately, the vast majority of us simply undergo the usual unattractive but benign course of chicken pox and then recover—but with zoster (chicken pox) virus sleeping latently in our deep nerve ganglia. Occasionally, the virus awakens and the resulting disease is "shingles."

Herpes Zoster: Pain and Scarring of Shingles

Shingles, known medically as herpes zoster, is an often painful and scarring disease. It is estimated that it causes five to ten percent of all infectious skin disease. Rarely, the disease follows exposure to someone with chicken pox or zoster, but almost always it is from reactivation of virus sleeping in your own nerve ganglion. What factors awaken the virus are as yet unknown, but once awake the viruses travel back down your nerve and cause what can be a massive eruption of blisters and swelling localized just to that area of your body fed by that particular nerve.

In their passage through your nerves, the viruses stir up much inflammation and irritation, thus causing pain which may be quite severe. Sometimes, in spite of the best treatment available, the inflammation of the nerves turns to permanent scarring and the pain becomes a long-term neuralgia. This neuralgia may feel like sharp shooting pains, severe gnawing dull pain, constant itching, or a crawly "wormy" feeling in the part of your body affected. It may be several months before your doctor knows if your pain will be permanent or will lessen with time.

In the skin, the zoster blisters and inflammation are much more severe than those caused by herpes simplex. Depending on which nerve ganglion is involved, you may have a rash running all the way down one leg, around one side of your chest, over one side of your head and involving your eye. Zoster almost never involves both sides of the body and, unlike herpes simplex, it almost never comes back again. It may, however, spread over your body like chicken pox. The blisters rupture within a few days, leaving a raw, red ulcerated area of skin. Thick crusts then form. When they finally peel off after two or three weeks, there is frequently a mild to moderate pitted scarring of the skin which will always mark the site of an attack of zoster.

Zoster and the Eye

If your fifth nerve ganglion is involved (see "Herpes and Our Eyes—Keratitis and Iritis"), the forehead, cheek and eye may sustain considerable damage. You may have severe, chronic pain, scarring of your skin, or paralysis of the muscles which open or move your eye. The eyeball itself may have scarring of its clear front window, the cornea, with loss of vision. Inflammation in the eye may cause glaucoma (raised eye pressure) or cataract (cloudy lens in your eye), both of which may take your sight. Zoster scarring of the eye is different from herpes simplex scarring, not in appearance but in the fact that your eye physician cannot operate on it to restore your sight by corneal transplant. Those zoster scarred eyes do not heal well after such surgery and your eye may be lost altogether if a transplant is attempted.

Treatment

Therapy of the skin ulcers is generally just good hygiene such as warm saltwater compresses. A clean facecloth soaked in warm salt water made with one teaspoon of table salt per quart of tap water is placed gently over the affected skin for five to ten minutes twice daily until the scabs fall off. This keeps the area clean and gets rid of dead tissue.

Pain during the first two weeks is handled by common drugs such as aspirin or aspirinlike compounds, or, if necessary, a short-term course of narcotics such as codeine or Percocet™. If after this time the pain is increasing or already severe and showing no signs of improving, your doctor may decide that you need two or three weeks of cortisone-type therapy. The purpose of using such an anti-inflammatory drug is to try to prevent permanent scarring of the inflamed nerves and thereby prevent permanent pain. This therapy is usually quite successful. Because the cortisone family does impair your body's ability to fight infections, your doctor may want to get a chest X ray and a few blood tests before starting treatment. These tests may be ordered, even if cortisone drugs are not to be given, as a safety precaution and part of your general examination.

Chronic pain or itch may develop in spite of all treatment. Fortunately, many patients get excellent relief simply by taking pills such as Triavil 2-10™ three or four times daily. Other drugs which are used with some success include the anticonvulsion drugs (to quiet the irritated nerves) such as Tegretol™ or Depakene™. In the rare cases where these drugs don't work, anesthesiologists may be called upon to inject the ganglion with chemicals such as alcohol. This kills the nerve and rids you of pain, but that part of your body then becomes completely numb. This may be better than constant pain, however. Other antipain treatments used by neurosurgeons include surgically destroying the nerve or the implantation of tiny electrodes which counter-stimulate the nerve and block the sending of pain messages to your brain.

Eye disease caused by zoster is a special problem. If ulcers on the front of your eye do not heal, a clear therapeutic soft contact lens may have to be placed on your eye by your physician. These lenses are left in place for several months while the ulcers heal underneath. Any glaucoma is usually treated with eye drops or pills and cataracts may be removed after your eye has quieted down. Paralysis of the muscles which move your eyes and lids almost always goes away completely after several months and treatment is not necessary or possible.

As a rule, specific antiviral therapy is not yet used against zoster—except in the most extreme cases. Nonetheless, medical science is moving rapidly toward developing good specific treatment for this infection, particularly in chronically ill (cancer) patients. The following case reports are some of the first examples of specific therapy by topical IDU or intravenous acyclovir or BVDU pills. For the most part, treatment was highly successful, although one case, you will see, persisted in recurrent attacks.

Specific Antiviral Treatment of Chicken Pox-Zoster Infections†

In our many attempts to find effective treatment for acute zoster infections, we have come across some rather unexpected results. The following case report taught us that treatment with some antiviral drugs in one part of the body may be very effective, while identical treatment of the same disease located elsewhere in your body may have little to no effect.[14]

Eighty patients with herpes zoster of the chest and forty-two patients with herpes zoster of the face were studied. Treatment was either the antiviral IDU in DMSO, DMSO‡ alone or salt water applied to the skin. The patients who had zoster infection of the face entered the study within two to three days of the onset of their disease, while those who had infection of the chest entered sooner, within one to two days. In addition, the facial zoster was associated with a more severe inflammation, the patients were more severely ill with high fevers and had a greater incidence of neurological problems. This neurological problem was characterized by severe neurologic pain and its occurrence related to the time of healing of the blisters. The longer the patient had zoster blisters, the greater the chance of having severe and prolonged pain even after healing had occurred.

When the results of the study were analyzed, it was found that the facial zoster had healed much more quickly than the chest infections, in spite of the fact that the facial infections

† See also "Therapy and Prevention of Genital Herpes."
‡ Not FDA-approved for drug use.

had been more severe to begin with. IDU had no effect at all on the rapidity of healing of the chest blisters nor on the duration of pain which lingered after healing occurred. IDU did, however, have a very significant effect on facial infection and improved the healing and reduced the duration of the pain markedly. Blood studies indicated that there were no bad side effects from the IDU-DMSO on either the liver or bone marrow (blood-making) function of the patients involved.

The above study indicates that we may expect a variety of responses to identical treatment of zoster infections and this variety is dependent on the location of the infection in your body. The physicians carrying out this work estimated that about 20 percent of the antiviral IDU was absorbed by their method of application and they suggested that other techniques of applying the drug might help to reduce the waste of the drug.

Until recently, chicken pox-zoster infection of the brain, meningitis and encephalitis, were felt to be largely due to an allergic reaction to the organism and not to true invasion of these tissues by the virus. We now know that in some patients, particularly children with such severe diseases as leukemia or cancer of the brain, may develop widespread infection with this virus, including infection of the brain and spinal cord. Fortunately, this too can now be successfully treated.[32]

Two children, one with acute leukemia and the other with cancer of the brain, developed widespread infection with chicken pox-zoster. Infection of the brain was confirmed by virus culture of their spinal fluid and blood tests confirmed that their white blood cell immune abilities were severely impaired. They were unable to mount a defense against this invading virus. Both children received treatment with acyclovir for five days intravenously. Within three days, the dreadfully ill children began to improve. Cultures of their blisters failed to grow out virus and the spinal fluid cultures were also negative for virus at the end of treatment. There was no sign of any toxic side effect from the drug and both children recovered from their attack of widespread herpes zoster infection.

As we have noted, antiviral treatment can often be very effective in speeding recovery from an acute attack of herpes simplex. Unfortunately, this treatment does not appear to have any effect on subsequent recurrences of the same form of herpes or perhaps a different member of that same family such as zoster. The following case report is an unusual example of a patient who was treated with several courses of different antiviral drugs and responded well to one of the drugs but could not be prevented from having recurrences of her illness once the drug was discontinued.[48]

> This woman had Hodgkin's lymphoma (cancer of the lymph glands) which had not responded well to treatment with X-ray or anticancer therapy. One day she was admitted to the hospital because of acute pain due to swelling of her genitalia and a band of blisters which ran from her lower back down into the groin and to her genitalia. A diagnosis of herpes zoster infection was made and the virus was grown out in tissue culture. She was put on treatment with vidarabine intravenously, but despite this therapy her zoster infection spread throughout her body. Vidarabine was stopped and, twelve days after the onset of her illness, she was given acyclovir intravenously for five days. Within a day and a half, the spreading of the blisters had stopped and healing had begun. Unfortunately, ten days after the acyclovir treatment had been discontinued, another crop of herpetic blisters appeared throughout her body. She was again treated with acyclovir, this time for ten days. Once again, the spread of blisters stopped and healing was complete.

As we can see from this patient's unfortunate course, acyclovir treatment does not wipe out latent zoster infection but is effective in controlling an acute attack. Because the virus blisters kept reappearing throughout her body, it was felt that the germs were spreading through her blood. Zoster, then, does not differ in its response to antiviral therapy from herpes simplex. Neither herpes virus can yet be eradicated from your body by antiviral treatment as it exists today, but we can do much to control the immediate infectious problems.

Severe herpes zoster infection can now also be treated with the new antiviral drug BVDU (bromovinyldeoxyuridine) when given as a *pill*.[12]

Three women and one man, ranging in age from forty-seven to sixty-eight years, developed severe herpes zoster infection. Three of these patients had an underlying disorder of cancer and one had hyperthyroidism. The zoster disease which they developed was severe involvement of the chest and widespread involvement of the entire body, neck, and eyes. BVDU pills were given four times daily for five days. Within one day, all new blister formation had stopped and the blisters which already existed healed rapidly. In the two patients who had widely spread zoster ulcers, fever was gone within twenty-four hours of starting treatment. At no time during therapy or afterward did any patient experience any uncomfortable side effects from their drugs.

The foregoing case shows how effective this new specific and nontoxic antiviral pill can be in controlling and healing severe herpes zoster infection. This pill is of use, of course, only in the acute infectious phase and would not be of help to patients who have gone through acute illness and are now suffering from the chronic pain known as postherpetic neuralgia. Unfortunately, the neuralgic pain is not due to virus persisting in the body but to scarring of the nerves which occurred during the acute illness. As I have discussed elsewhere, there are other modes of treating the pain caused from herpetic neuralgia.

19. THE GAY POPULATION AND HERPETIC INFECTIONS

Herpes simplex type-1 and type-2 and zoster infections are no different in incidence, severity, or management in the gay population than those infections occurring in the heterosexual population. *All earlier discussions and suggestions for protection apply to gay and straight people alike.* There is, however, another herpes virus which is causing severe problems which are largely confined to the gay population. It appears to be a venereal illness.

In mid-1981, the medical world first became alerted to an epidemic of chronic and potentially lethal herpes virus infection associated in a number of cases with a malignant tumor know as Kaposi's sarcoma. The Centers for Disease Control in Atlanta (CDC) is now analyzing more than one hundred and sixty case reports, with five to six new cases coming in each week.

The final results from these and other studies are not yet in, but a number of important features have already been recognized. The patients are usually young homosexual men living in large cities. Many of them use drugs, particularly "poppers" (amylnitrate or butyrlnitrate), which are commonly inhaled for the purpose of intensifying orgasm.

While many bacteria have been shown to cause severe disease in these young men, the germs which stand out as highly suspect in starting the entire disease are the herpes viruses, cytomegalovirus (CMV) and herpes simplex virus type-2. CMV infection is the most common binding factor among cases reported thus far. It is well known that this herpes virus is passed in breast milk in one out of four nursing mothers who have CMV infection themselves. CMV infection is particularly common in the homosexual community, with more than nine out of every ten men having evidence of the infection. Only five out of every ten heterosexual men have evidence of CMV. We know that this virus can persist both in the semen and in the urine for many months and thus serve as the source not only of first infection but many reinfections with the same organism in sexual partners.

But what does CMV do to cause chronic infectious disease and cancer? CMV is particularly effective at interfering with our body's ability to fight infection. Specifically, this virus causes a marked reduction in numbers of and interference with the function of the white blood cells which normally fight infection. The natural killer cells are almost totally wiped out and those which persist are rendered ineffective. Such interference with the body's immune defense mechanisms then allows other organisms, such as herpes simplex virus or bacterial infections, to spread throughout the body. Similarly, just as the body cannot fight infections, it can not fight malignant changes which lead to the development of a particular form of cancer known as sarcoma.

Until the present epidemic, Kaposi's sarcoma was a rare malignant tumor found almost exclusively among the elderly in the United States. The disease is more commonly found in equatorial Africa among all age groups. Kaposi's sarcoma appears on the skin or mucous membranes as bluish, violaceous, or brownish nodules. In elderly Americans, it may be fatal over an eight-to-thirteen-year period, but the sarcoma being found in the homosexual population is behaving more like that found in African patients. Many of those men afflicted have died from the sarcoma within just three to twenty months, a most rampant and unusual course probably due, in great part, to the paralysis of the blood cell immune defense system in these people. In general, however, *these tumors may respond well to early X-ray therapy.*

The following case reports are included to give you some familiarity with the severity of this illness and the need to seek early medical attention, both to ensure early diagnosis and early aggressive therapy.[19]

Case 1: Patient number one was a thirty-three-year-old homosexual man who had been entirely healthy until he developed a fever and swollen glands in his neck. After six months of recurring fevers and chronic fungal infection of his skin, he was admitted to a major medical center. Examination at that time revealed a generalized loss of hair, moist superficial ulcers of his buttocks, fungal infection of his mouth (thrush), and ulcerating sores at the end of his index fingers.

CMV was cultured from his urine and herpes simplex from his throat, perianal area, and fingertip ulcers.

Intensive treatment with a new antifungal agent resulted in marked improvement in the sores on his buttocks and fingertips, but his fever continued. He was given five days of intravenous treatment with the antiviral drug acyclovir and herpes simplex virus could no longer be recovered from the buttocks, throat, or fingertips. CMV, however, was still present in his urine.

He was discharged but readmitted one month later because
of difficulty breathing, cough, and fever. The sores on his
fingers and around his rectum were nearly healed, but a
pneumonia was present. Herpes simplex virus was cultured
from the lung washings and blood tests showed severe
depression of his body's ability to fight infection, due to the
depression of his white blood cells. He was given intensive
treatment with antibiotics and acyclovir but remained chronically ill.

Case 2: Patient number two was a thirty-three-year-old
homosexual man who was admitted to a major medical center with a four-month history of daily fevers and feeling generally ill. Blood tests showed a generalized depression of the
white blood cells which fight infection. CMV was cultured
from his urine and blood.

Several days later, he developed rectal and oral fungal infections and became acutely ill. He was treated intensively
with antibiotics for a bacterial pneumonia and recovered.

Four months later, he was readmitted for recurrent pneumonia and CMV was cultured from a lung biopsy specimen.
He recovered after four weeks of intensive antibiotic therapy
and was discharged, taking low-dose antibiotics as a preventive measure against recurrent infection.

Case 3: Patient number three was a thirty-year-old previously healthy homosexual man who was admitted to a
major medical center because of one month of pain on
swallowing and fungal infection of his mouth. Blood tests
showed a marked decrease in his white blood cell count.

He was treated with antifungal drugs with improvement
and was discharged only to be readmitted five days later with
fever, shortness of breath, and cough. He had a bacterial
pneumonia which responded to intensive antibiotic therapy.

Two months later, he was readmitted because of severe
difficulty in swallowing. A biopsy of the ulcers seen in his
upper digestive tract (esophagus) grew out CMV. He improved on treatment with antifungal agents. Two months

later, he again had bacterial pneumonia, which responded well to antibiotic treatment. CMV was cultured from his urine and a lung biopsy.

Three months later, a purple slightly elevated plaquelike lesion with a central nodule appeared on the left wall of his chest. He had three similar plaques in his upper digestive tract. Biopsies of these areas revealed Kaposi's sarcoma.

Case 4: Patient number four was a thirty-two-year-old homosexual man who developed perianal blistering. Biopsy suggested CMV infection. Five months later, he developed fever, loss of appetite, weight loss, pain in his abdomen, and rectal bleeding. Four months later, he had further rectal bleeding. He was admitted to a major medical center, at which time it was noted that the perianal ulcer had spread across the buttocks and cultures were positive for herpes simplex type-2 and CMV. Blood tests revealed depression of the white cell count. The patient, who was treated with vidarabine and subsequently with acyclovir with no effect, continued to be chronically ill.

The following case reports describe homosexual men who developed gradually enlarging herpes simplex type-2 ulcers around the anus. These men also had CMV, bacterial and fungal infection associated with a poor body white blood cell defense system. One responded to antiviral treatment; the other, unfortunately, did not.[40]

Case 1: Patient number one was a twenty-eight-year-old homosexual man who developed a dull pain in his lower stomach region and rectal bleeding. The diagnosis of perianal abscess was made and he was treated surgically. One month later, he developed fever and weight loss and, after additional anal surgery, developed a perianal ulcer which gradually spread across his buttocks. He was treated intensively with antibiotic and anti-inflammatory drugs, but his fever and perianal ulcers persisted.

He was admitted to a major medical center because of extreme weight loss and further spread of the ulcer. Cultures from the ulcerated buttocks grew herpes simplex type-2 and he was treated successively with the antiviral drugs, vidarabine, interferon, and FIAC without success.

Case 2: Patient number two was a twenty-two-year-old homosexual man who developed fever and night sweats, followed by a gradual loss of weight. Six months later, he developed blistering lesions around his rectum and cultures grew out herpes simplex type-2. He suffered spiking fevers, sleepiness, loss of appetite, and continued weight loss. The perianal ulcers gradually enlarged and he then developed similar lesions around his nose and mouth.

He was treated with intensive antifungal and antibiotic agents. Therapy with the antiviral vidarabine did not affect his herpes infection, but acyclovir treatment for ten days resulted in gradual healing of the perianal and facial ulcers.

Three months later, the herpes ulcers recurred and virus was again cultured from the lesions. He was successfully treated with acyclovir. At this time, however, blue nodules were noted on the back and shaft of his penis. Biopsy revealed a diagnosis of Kaposi's sarcoma.

The foregoing case reports are distressing indeed and a source of great concern to the gay community. As both CMV and homosexuality are surely as old as time itself, we can only ask why now and why this particular population? The disease syndrome in fact, is not confined entirely to the gay community but has now been reported among heterosexual drug abusers. What is the common bond? It appears to be depression of the body's white blood cells, the immune defense system against infection. In the case of the gay population, this appears to be largely due to infection with CMV, which has most likely been transmitted venereally. If a homosexual man has many sexual partners, he is more at risk for contracting venereal disease through continuous reinfection with more CMV via semen. Lesbians are not prone to having multiple sexual partners nor is an ejaculate involved. This difference in social patterns appears to have spared the lesbian community from the frightening epidemic now spreading through the homosexual community. Currently, among the patients with this illness, only one woman is known to the Centers for Disease Control.

One may hypothesize, then, that CMV is passed from man to man via the shedding of virus through semen and urine. *Use of condoms during sexual activity would, in theory, minimize this virus transmission. An indiscriminate sex life or drug use is not a requirement for contracting this illness, however.* In the cases reported earlier, one patient was highly active sexually and frequented gay bars and bathhouses, a second had lived for seven years with just one partner, and the third patient had had several partners, all of whom were regular and known to him.[19] In none of these three men was there any history of illicit drug exposure.

As so many causative factors seem to vary, we can only guess, in our present state of knowledge, as to the mechanism behind this disease characterized by chronic infection and the occasional development of malignant disease. It seems possible that the existence of chronic viral infection such as CMV, plus or minus drug use such as poppers may, in certain men, cause an inhibition of their bodies' white blood cell system and thus, an inhibition of the immune surveillance system which defends against infection and cancer. The patients start out with a mild nonspecific illness such as fungal infection of the mouth. But as the white blood cell defect becomes more severe, more serious infections take over and the body is unable to defend itself. In addition, the sarcoma, whatever its cause (and it may be CMV-induced), is free to grow because the body cannot defend itself against cancerous cells. The end result is a severely ill patient who has multiple infections and possible cancerous changes on the skin or mucous membranes of his body.

At the moment, we can only advise patients who develop any of the symptoms described in the case reports to seek early medical help. This will not only assure you of early therapy, but aid your physician in determining the cause and subsequent prevention of spread of this illness.

Note: The illness described above is similar to Acquired Immune Deficiency Syndrome (AIDS), which has received recent widespread publicity. AIDS is currently considered an illness of unknown cause. Approximately 75 percent of the patients who have it, however, are homosexual, and 25 percent are drug addicts.

20. HOPE FOR THE FUTURE

Antiviral Drugs for Genital, Skin, Mouth, and Eye Infections*

Until recently, all antiviral drugs developed were too toxic to be given systematically (by pill or injection), except in life-threatening situations, such as in brain infections. The drugs were also of no use on the skin or in relieving genital herpes and certainly nothing reached the source of recurrent infections, the deep nerve ganglia. We only had therapy for the eye. Now scientists have developed at least two drugs, ACV (acyclovir, Zovirax™) and BVDU (bromovinyldeoxyuridine), which appear to be effective in treating many forms of herpes. Human studies are still being carried out on ACV in the United States and Europe and on BVDU in Europe. The ACV trials are further along than those of BVDU, but both drugs look very good.

What is unique about these medications, compared to the older drugs, is that they are activated only by herpes virus enzymes. This means that the drugs are active only in cells which actually contain virus and pass by all normal cells. Such a specific site of action makes these medications relatively nontoxic.

ACV has been shown in the laboratory to be very effective against both type-1 and type-2 herpes simplex and against chicken pox-zoster (shingles) virus. The first studies on humans have shown that it is successful when given intravenously to treat herpes simplex pneumonia (usually fatal), widespread skin infection in children with leukemia, herpes simplex of the mouth and throat, chicken pox (zoster virus) pneumonia, and shingles. When used as an ointment, it rapidly cures herpes simplex ulcers of the eye.

In studies of ACV ointment therapy of genital infections, it has been shown that patients suffering a first attack have a much shorter period of pain, itching, and shedding of infectious virus

* See also "Therapy and Prevention of Genital Herpes."

compared to untreated patients. In patients with recurrent genital infections, the period of shedding of infectious virus was shortened and the number of new blisters notably reduced in ACV-treated patients when compared to those people without treatment.

Similarly, in studies of ACV ointment therapy of herpes skin infections, the amount of infectious virus was reduced, although there was not much effect on the disease itself. In these last studies, it was felt that earlier application of treatment might have produced better results. As discussed in greater detail earlier in this book, acyclovir has just been FDA-approved for marketing for treatment of primary genital infections and skin herpes in the chronically ill patient.

ACV may also be given by mouth (as a powder or pill), with good therapeutic levels of drug appearing in the blood. There were no notable toxic side effects when the drug was given orally, as an ointment, or intravenously. All of these studies are most encouraging and larger ones are now under way.

BVDU is also activated just by herpes virus enzymes and is nontoxic, while being very effective in treating herpes infections. The first human studies using ointment in the eye indicate that it works very well. BVDU pills were very effective in treatment of acute severe zoster in recent studies and laboratory evidence indicates that future work on other forms of herpes in humans will also be successful. It is more effective against type-1 than type-2 herpes but because nearly one third of all genital herpes infections in people under age twenty-five are due to type-1 this drug has obvious potential for treatment in this area.

The new technology of using recombinant DNA techniques (genetic engineering) for the inexpensive and mass production of drugs such as insulin has also made the antiviral, interferon, available in plentiful supply. This "natural protein" is produced by our own bodies in response to viral invasion of any kind and contributes significantly to our recovery from many viral illnesses. Herpes viruses of many types are susceptible to interferon if only the correct dosage can be given for an adequate period of time. Many studies on the use of interferon for treating illnesses—from herpes to certain forms of cancer—are now under way and preliminary results in a number of them are encouraging. We must wait for further information before we know precisely how this drug should be used, but it is at least one more weapon in the antiviral armamentarium.

Other new antivirals, such as FIAC, are discussed briefly in "Therapy and Prevention of Genital Herpes." We should all be encouraged by the progress now being made in government and privately supported research laboratories. Many new antivirals, such as those already discussed, are being produced and studied intensively. They represent just one approach to herpes. Vaccines are another.

Vaccines

This method of treatment has not worked well in the past, but there is now a new theory of how herpes works. It is felt by some experts that there are many kinds of herpes simplex type-1 and type-2. Some of these are "good" viruses and some are "bad."

If you are lucky, you will be infected with "good" virus the first time around. Good viruses travel to the deep nerve ganglia and go to sleep, but they never wake up again to cause another attack of herpes. But the best effect of having a "good" virus already in your ganglia is that it will block a "bad" virus from ever getting in. You are protected for life. Unfortunately, some of the viruses are "bad," however. This means that they travel to your ganglia during your first attack and then stay there in a cycle of sleep and frequent waking up to cause many attacks of herpes. It is unlikely that vaccines made from "good" but alive virus which could travel to your ganglia will ever be given because of the possible association of herpes with cancer. But scientists using recombinant DNA technology are learning more and more about which parts of the viral genetic substance do what. One day they may be able to create a herpes virus vaccine which is missing the part of the gene that may be related to cancer but has the part that keeps it forever asleep in your ganglion and protects you from infection with a similar but "bad" herpes virus. Laboratory studies on these new vaccines are under way and human studies are just a few years away.

21. GETTING INTO NEW TREATMENT STUDIES

You may often read about new treatments for herpes and wonder why your own physician cannot offer them to you. This is because all new drugs to be considered for sale in this country must undergo thorough study to assure that they work and are safe before the Food and Drug Administration will approve them. To do otherwise would mean that many useless and possibly unsafe treatments would be sold and many people could be hurt. Most people probably think about the thalidomide disaster in Europe each time they see a child without arms or legs.

The study of new drugs in the United States is done in humans only after laboratory work has shown that it is effective and safe enough to be tried with patients. The first place such work is done is usually in large medical centers affiliated with a university medical school. Only after many patients (usually hundreds) have been treated are investigators outside of the hospital-medical center allowed to use the drug. This is after the first studies have been well analyzed and the drug shown to be safe and to work.

Therefore, if you wish to be involved in receiving some of the newer treatments for herpes, it is best to contact a major university medical school hospital and ask to speak to a doctor in the department that would be studying your kind of infection. If you have genital herpes, you would call either the department of gynecology (women) or urology (men). Dermatology (skin) or infectious disease departments also often take care of genital infections, so it is worth trying them whether your infection is genital or skin. If you have it in the mouth, dental schools often take care of herpes infections and are worth calling. For the eye, call ophthalmology.

When you call, either mention the name of a specific drug you have heard of to see if they are studying it or, if they are not, ask if they can tell you where it is being studied or who the sponsor (usually a drug company) is. You may then go on to contact them.

If you have no particular treatment in mind, you can volunteer yourself for a new study that might be going on in the center you call. Remember, however, that studies are limited to just a few medical centers across the country.

Before placing you in a study, the doctors must decide whether you would be a suitable candidate for the treatment and might stand to benefit from it. Sometimes they are not always working on your particular form of infection but can put you on a list if such a study is started in the future. The doctors must also tell you what the treatment is, what the risks and benefits are, how long you might be in the study, and how often you must be examined and how. They will ask you to sign a consent sheet telling you much of this if you do enter the study. You are also free to discontinue being in the study at any time, for any reason, without obligation. As new and better forms of treatment come along, it is often worth exploring becoming a member of such a study group.

EPILOGUE

Herpes viruses have been with us since time immemorial, living with us in an almost symbiotic relationship. But the social revolution of the 1960s changed our lives and our ways of loving each other. With that change, some of the herpes viruses changed too. They changed not only their usual sites of residence in our bodies but the frequency with which we found them in unexpected locations. We were all caught off guard. An epidemic of genital infections began more than a decade ago but because many people were afraid to talk about it or to seek help, the medical profession was unable to respond, either in terms of medical or emotional support and advice.

When the enormity of the problem was eventually recognized just a very few years ago, everyone became involved in a process of catching up. The medical profession, federal agencies, and the pharmaceutical industry all had to learn more about herpes as quickly as possible. We had to learn more about the illnesses this virus family caused so that we could advise patients as to how they could protect themselves from herpes or how to live successfully with it. We had to learn more about the basic biochemical nature of the viruses so that we could devise new drugs to interfere with the virus life cycle without interfering with the normal biochemical functions of our own bodies. But most of all, we had —and still have—to learn that having herpes is nothing of which we should be ashamed or frightened. Not knowing what to do, when to do it, and how to do it has been our worst enemy in coping with this virus. Hearing and seeing but not really knowing about something that affects so many of us on a very personal level can be terrifying. The emotional reactions to genital herpes have superceded the physical aspects of the infection.

But thousands upon thousands of people with this illness have come to terms with it and learned or taught themselves how to cope successfully with it. Emotional support groups have been formed all over the country and the medical profession and pharmaceutical industry have responded both by working out many of the do's and don'ts of herpetic infection and by developing and testing new and increasingly more effective therapy.

We are now in an era when not enough information is available and there is much confusion in the general population about which herpes virus does what. "Having herpes" in itself means little. Almost everyone in the country has one or more kinds of herpes virus living quietly, or not so quietly, in them. To dispel fear and to cope successfully with this common germ, we must know not just which herpes viruses we have but what behavioral pattern we can expect from them. Only then can we appreciate how rare or how harmless most forms of herpes illness are—and what we can do to minimize or protect ourselves from those forms which potentially could cause real problems. There is so much that can already be done to control the effects herpes has had on our lives. We can master it; it must not master us. It is simply a matter of learning a few new "rules and regulations" with which we can all live. We can make love safely, we can have babies safely, and no one need be alone in living with any form of herpes. Sympathetic and understanding emotional support groups and effective forms of treatment and prevention are available today—and tomorrow holds the promise of yet greater advances on all fronts in our efforts toward successfully "living with herpes."

CLINICAL CASES AND STUDIES CITED

1. Adam, E., et al., "Persistence of Virus-Shedding in Asymptomatic Women After Recovery from Herpes Genitalis," *Obstetrics and Gynecology* 54:171, 1979.

2. Aronson, M., et al., "Vidarabine Therapy for Severe Herpesvirus Infections," *Journal of the American Medical Association* 235:1339, 1976.

3. Becker, W., "The Epidemiology of Herpes Virus Infection in Three Racial Communities in Cape Town," *South African Medical Journal* 40:109, 1966.

4. Block, B., et al., "False Positive Amniotic Fluid Cytology in a Parturient with Active Genital Herpes Infection at Term," *Obstetrics and Gynecology* 54:658, 1979.

5. Borg, I., et al., "Herpes Simplex Virus as a Cause of Peptic Ulcer," *Scandinavian Journal of Gastroenterology* 15 (Suppl. 63):56, 1980.

6. Burnet, F., et al., "Herpes Simplex: A New Point of View," *Medical Journal of Australia* 26:637, 1939.

7. Bryson, Y., et al., "Successful Treatment of Initial Genital Herpes Simplex Virus Infection with Oral Acyclovir," *Clinical Research* 30:128a, 1982.

8. Chang, T., "Local Dissemination of Herpes Simplex Following Soaking or Sitz Bathing," *American Journal of Obstetrics and Gynecology* 131:343, 1978.

9. Corey, L., et al., "A Trial of Topical Acyclovir in Genital Herpes Simplex Virus Infections," *New England Journal of Medicine* 306:1313, 1982.

10. Curry, J., et al., "Proctitis Associated with Herpes Virus Hominis Type II Infection," *Canadian Medical Association Journal* 119:485, 1978.

11. Deardourff, S., et al., "Association Between Herpes Hominis Type II and the Male Genital Urinary Tract," *Journal of Urology* 112:126, 1974.

12. DeClercq, E., et al., "Oral (E)-5-(2-Bromovinyl)-2-Deoxyuridine in Severe Herpes Zoster," *British Medical Journal* 281:1178, 1980.

13. Dunkle, L., et al., "Neonatal Herpes Simplex Infection Possibly Acquired via Maternal Breast Milk," *Pediatrics* 63:250, 1979.

14. Esman, V., "Idoxuridine for Herpes Zoster," *Lancet,* p. 474, August 30, 1980.

15. Felman, Y., et al., "Herpes Simplex Virus Infections," *New York State Journal of Medicine* 79:179, 1979.

16. Fishbein, P., et al., "Herpes Simplex Esophagitis: A Cause of Upper Gastrointestinal Bleeding," *American Journal of Digestive Diseases* 24:540, 1979.

17. Francis, D., et al., "Nosocomial and Maternally Acquired Herpes Virus Hominis Infections," *American Journal of Diseases of Children* 130:889, 1975.

18. Golden, S., et al., "Disseminated Herpes Simplex Neonatorum," *American Journal of Obstetrics and Gynecology* 129:917, 1977.

19. Gottlieb, M., et al., "Pneumoncystis Carinii Pneumonia and Mucosal Candidiasis in Previously Healthy Homosexual Men," *New England Journal of Medicine* 305:1425, 1981.

20. Hinthorn, D., et al., "Recurrent Conjugal Neuralgia Caused by Herpes Virus Hominis Type II," *Journal of the American Medical Association* 236:587, 1976.

21. Hovig, D., et al., "Herpes Virus Homonis (Simplex) Infection with Recurrences During Infancy," *American Journal of Diseases of Children* 115:438, 1968.

22. Hutchinson, D., et al., "Congenital Herpetic Keratitis," *Archives of Ophthalmology* 93:70, 1975.

23. Jacobs, E., "Anal Infections Caused by Herpes Simplex Virus," *Diseases of the Colon and Rectum* 19:151, 1976.

24. Kaufman, R., et al., "Extragenital Type II Herpes Virus Infection," *American Journal of Obstetrics and Gynecology* 112:866, 1972.

25. Kaufman, R., et al., "Herpes Virus-Induced Antigens in the Squamous Cell Carcinoma in Situ of the Vulva," *New England Journal of Medicine* 305:483, 1981.

26. Kibrick, S., et al., "Pathogenesis of Infection with Herpes Simplex Virus with Special Reference to Nervous Tissue. Slow Latent and Temporate Virus Infection," *Monography* 2:143, 1965.

27. King, R., "Herpes Simplex Encephalitis in Pregnancy," *American Journal of Obstetrics and Gynecology* 135:1114, 1979.

28. Knox, S., et al., "Historical Findings in Subjects from a High Socioeconomic Group Who Have Genital Infections with Herpes Simplex Virus," *Sexually Transmitted Diseases* 9:15, 1982.

29. Langvad, A., et al., "Herpes Generalisata Infantum," *Danish Medical Bulletin* 10:153, 1963.

30. Luby, J., "Therapy in Genital Herpes," *New England Journal of Medicine* 306:1356, 1982.

31. Meister, F., Jr., et al., "Primary Herpetic Gingivostomatitis Accompanying Lesions on Fingers," *Journal of Oral Surgery* 37:508, 1979.

32. Nelson, T., et al., "Acyclovir for the Treatment of the Culture Positive Varicella-Zoster Meningoencephalitis," *Clinical Research* 28(5):855A, December 1983.

33. Owensby, L., et al., "Esophagitis Associated with Herpes Simplex Infection in an Immunocompetent Host," *Gastroenterology* 74:1305, 1978.

34. Pavan-Langston, D., Personal case records, 1982.

35. Peutherer, J., et al., "Necrotizing Balanitis Due to a Generalized Primary Infection with Herpes Simplex Virus Type II," *British Journal of Venereal Disease* 55:48, 1979.

36. Polayes, I., et al., "Treatment of Herpetic Whitlow," *Plastic and Reconstructive Surgery* 65:811, 1980.

37. Reeves, W., et al., "Risk of Recurrence After First Episodes of Genital Herpes," *New England Journal of Medicine* 305:315, 1981.

38. Shelley, W., "Herpetic Arthritis Associated with Disseminated Herpes Simplex in a Wrestler," *British Journal of Dermatology* 103:209, 1980.

39. Shortsleeve, M., et al., "Herpetic Esophagitis," *Diagnostic Radiology* 141:611, 1981.

40. Siegal, F., "Severe Acquired Immuno-Deficiency in Male Homosexual Manifested by Chronic Perianal Ulcerative Herpes Simplex Lesions," *New England Journal of Medicine* 305:1439, 1981.

41. Skoldenberg, B., et al., "Herpes Simplex Virus Type II in Acute Aseptic Meningitis," *British Medical Journal* 611, June 9, 1975.

42. Smith, J., et al., "The Incidence of Herpes Virus Hominis Antibodies in the Population," *Journal of Hygiene* 65:395, 1967.

43. Springer, D., et al., "A Syndrome of Acute Self-limiting Ulcerative Esophagitis in Young Adult, Probably Due to Herpes Simplex Virus," *American Journal of Digestive Diseases* 24:535, 1979.

44. Spence, M., "Inapparent Sexual Transmission of Herpes Simplex Virus Type II with Subsequent Fetal Death," *American Journal of Obstetrics and Gynecology* 130:591, 1978.

45. Spruance, S., "Antiviral Treatment of Recurrent Herpes Simplex Labialis Should Be Started Within Eight Hours After Lesion Onset," *Clinical Research* 30:100A, 1982.

46. Tear, E., et al., "Acyclovir for Suspected Systemic Herpes Infection," *Lancet* 42, January 5, 1980.

47. Van Der Mer, J., et al., "Acyclovir Therapy of Varicella-Zoster," *Lancet*, p. 473, August 30, 1980.

48. Von Schulthess, G., et al., "Acyclovir and Herpes Zoster," *New England Journal of Medicine* 305:1349, 1981.

49. Wheeler, C., Jr., et al., "Epidemic Cutaneous Herpes Simplex in Wrestlers (Herpes Gladiatorum)," *Journal of the American Medical Association* 194:145, 1965.

50. Young, E., et al., "Disseminated Herpes Virus Infection: Association with Primary Genital Herpes in Pregnancy," *Journal of the American Medical Association* 235:2731, 1976.

BIBLIOGRAPHY FOR FURTHER READING

GENERAL REVIEW ARTICLES and BOOKS

1. Garfield, E., "Herpes Simplex Virus Infection," Current Contents, p. 5, Part I, June 22, 1981; p. 5, Part II, June 29, 1981.

2. Juel-Jensen, B., and Maccallum, F., Herpes Simplex Varicella and Zoster. Philadelphia: J. B. Lippincott Co., 1972 (194 pages).

3. Juretic, M., Herpetic Infections of Man. Hanover, N.H.: University Press of New England, 1980 (201 pages).

4. Overall, J., "Persistent Problems with Persistent Herpes Viruses," New England Journal of Medicine 305:95, 1981.

5. Rand, K., "Herpes Simplex Virus: Clinical Syndromes and Current Therapy," Comprehensive Therapy 8:44, 1982.

GENITAL HERPES SIMPLEX

6. Amstey, M., "Genital Herpesvirus Infection," Clinical Obstetrics and Gynecology 1889, 1975.

7. Belsey, E., et al., "Current Approaches to the Diagnosis of Herpes Genitalis," British Journal of Venereal Disease 54:115, 1978.

8. Blough, H., et al., "Successful Treatment of Human Genital Herpes Infections with 2-deoxy-D-glucose," Journal of the American Medical Association 241:2798, 1979.

9. Chang, T., et al., "Treatment with Levamisole of Recurrent Herpes Genitalis," Antimicrobial Agents and Chemotherapy 13:809, 1978.

10. Corey, L., et al., "Clinical Course of Genital Herpes: Implications for Therapeutic Trials," in The Human Herpesviruses, ed. A. Nahmias et al. New York: Elsevier Co., 1981, p. 496.

11. Corey, L., et al., "Topical Therapy of Genital Herpes Simplex Virus Infections with Acyclovir," Antimicrobial Agents and Chemotherapy. Chicago, November 4–6, 1981, number 31 (abstract 21st Interscience Conference).

12. Crumpacker, C., et al., "Resistance of Herpes Simplex Virus to Acycloguanosine," Virology 105:171, 1980.

13. Goodheart, G., "Treatment of Genital Herpes Simplex," New England Journal of Medicine 300:1338, 1979.

14. Kalinyk, J., et al., "Incidence and Distribution of Herpes Simplex Virus Type I and II from Genital Lesions in College Women," Journal of Medical Virology 1:175, 1977.

15. Kaufman, R., et al., "Clinical Features of Herpes Genitalis," Cancer Research 33:1446, 1978.

16. Nahmias, A., et al., "Herpes Simplex Viruses I and II—Basic and Clinical Aspects," *Disease a Month,* Yearbook Med. Pub. 25:1, 1979.

17. Nahmias, A., et al., "Type II Herpes Simplex Virus Infections," *Survey of Ophthalmology* 21:115, 1976.

18. Nasemann, T., et al., "Vaccination for Herpes Simplex Genitalis," *British Journal of Venereal Disease* 55:121, 1979.

19. Overall, J., Jr., "Antiviral Chemotherapy of Oral and Genital Herpes Simplex Virus Infection," in *The Human Herpesviruses,* ed. A. Nahmias et al., New York: Elsevier Co., 1981, p. 446.

20. Person, D., et al., "Herpes Virus Type II in Genital Urinary Tract Infections," *American Journal of Obstetrics and Gynecology* 116:993, 1973.

21. Reeves, W., et al., "Risk of Recurrence After First Episodes of Genital Herpes," *New England Journal of Medicine* 305:315, 1981.

22. Rosenthal, M., "Genital Herpes Simplex Virus Infections," *Primary Care* 6:517, 1979.

23. Singh, B., et al., "Virucidal Effect of Certain Chemical Contraceptives on Type II Herpesvirus," *American Journal of Obstetrics and Gynecology* 126:422, 1976.

24. Stone, W., "Atypical Herpesvirus Hominis Type II Infection in Uremic Patients Receiving Immunosuppressive Therapy," *American Journal of Medicine* 63:511, 1976.

25. Vontver, L., et al., "Clinical Course and Diagnosis of Genital Herpes Simplex Infection and Evaluation of Topical Surfactant Therapy," *American Journal of Obstetrics and Gynecology* 133:548, 1979.

26. Yen, S., et al., "Herpes Simplex Infection in Female Genital Tract," *American Journal of Obstetrics and Gynecology* 25:479, 1965.

RECTAL HERPES INFECTION
27. Curry, J., et al., "Proctitis Associated with Herpes Virus Hominis Type II Infection," *Kansas Medical Association Journal* 119:485, 1978.

28. Goldmeier, D., "Proctitis and Herpes Simplex Virus in Homosexual Men," *British Journal of Venereal Disease* 56:111, 1980.

PREGNANCY AND POSTDELIVERY CARE
29. Hatherley, L., et al., "Herpesvirus in an Obstetric Hospital," *Medical Journal of Australia* 2: Part 1, 205, Part 2, 273, Part 3, 325, 1980.

30. Kejani, N., et al., "Subclinical Herpes Simplex Genitalis Infections in the Perinatal Period," *American Journal of Obstetrics and Gynecology* 135:547, 1979.

31. Kibrick, S., "Herpes Simplex in Breast Milk," *Pediatrics* 64:390, 1979.

32. Kibrick, S., "Herpes Simplex Infection at Term, What to Do with Mother, Newborn and Nursery Personnel," *Journal of the American Medical Association* 243:157, 1980.

33. Kobbermann, T., "Maternal Death Secondary to Disseminated Herpesvirus Hominis," *American Journal of Obstetrics and Gynecology* 137:742, 1980.

34. Schreiner, R., et al., "Maternal Oral Herpes: Isolation Policy," *Pediatrics* 63:247, 1979.

35. Whitley, R., et al., "Vidarabine Therapy of Neonatal Herpes Simplex Viral Infection," *Pediatrics* 66:495, 1980.

CANCER
36. Schwartz, P., et al., "Type II Herpes Simplex Virus and Vulvar Carcinoma in Situ," *New England Journal of Medicine* 305:517, 1981.

37. Stern, J., "Herpesvirus-Induced Antigen in Squamous Cell Carcinoma in Situ of the Vulva," *New England Journal of Medicine* 305:1586, 1981.

ORAL, FACIAL, AND EYE HERPES INFECTIONS
38. Bader, C., et al., "Natural History of Recurrent Facial-Oral Infection with Herpes Simplex Virus," *Journal of Infectious Disease* 138:897, 1978.

39. Duckworth, R., "Oral Herpes Simplex Virus Infection," *Journal of the Royal Society of Medicine* 72:126, 1979.

40. Frick, J., "Infectious Disease Hazard," *North Carolina Dental Journal*, p. 10, January 1973.

41. Pavan-Langston, D. (author/editor), *Ocular Viral Disease*, International Ophthalmology Clinics. Boston: Little, Brown & Co., 1975 (275 pages).

42. Pavan-Langston, D. (author/editor), *Manual of Ocular Diagnosis and Therapeutics*, Boston: Little, Brown & Co., 1980 (479 pages).

43. Pavan-Langston, D., "Clinical Evaluation of Ara-A and IDU in Treatment of Ocular Herpes," *American Journal of Ophthalmology* 80:495, 1975.

44. Pavan-Langston, D., "Major Ocular Viral Infections," in *Antivirals in Medicine*, ed. G. Galasso, T. Merigan, and R. Buchanan. New York: Raven Press, 1979, p. 253.

45. Pavan-Langston, D., "Ocular Herpetic Disease: Simplex and Zoster," in *Diseases of the Cornea*, ed. G. Smolin and R. Thoft. Boston: Little, Brown & Co., 1982.

46. Pavan-Langston, D., et al., "Trifluorothymidine (Trifluridine) and Idoxuridine Therapy of Ocular Herpes," *American Journal of Ophthalmology* 84:818, 1977.

47. Pavan-Langston, D., et al., "Acyclic Antimetabolite (Acyclovir) Therapy of Experimental Herpes Simplex Keratitis," *American Journal of Ophthalmology* 86:618, 1978.

48. Pavan-Langston, D., et al., "Ganglionic Herpes Simplex and Systemic Acyclovir," *Archives of Ophthalmology* 99:1417, 1981.

49. Pavan-Langston, D., et al., "Acyclovir and Vidarabine in the Treatment of Ulcerative Herpes Simplex Keratitis," *American Journal of Ophthalmology* 92:829, 1981.

50. Spruance, S., et al., "Natural History of Recurrent Herpes Simplex Labialis," *New England Journal of Medicine* 297:69, 1977.

ANTIVIRAL DRUGS AND OTHER THERAPY

51. Burns, W., et al., "Acyclovir-Resistant Herpes Simplex After Intravenous Treatment," *Lancet* 1:421, 1982.

52. DeClercq, E., "Nucleoside Analogues as Antiviral Agents," *Acta Microbiologica of the Academy of Science,* Hungary 28:289, 1981.

53. Field, H., et al., "Recurrent Herpes Simplex: The Outlook for Systemic Antiviral Agents," *British Medical Journal* 282:1821, 1981.

54. Guinan, M., et al., "Topical Ether and Herpes Simplex Labialis," *Journal of the American Medical Association* 243:1059, 1980.

55. Hirsch, M., et al., "Drug Therapy: Antiviral Agents," *New England Journal of Medicine* 302: (16)903 and 302:(17)949, 1980.

56. Maudgal, P., et al., "Efficacy of BVDU in Topical Treatment of Herpes Simplex Keratitis," *Archives Klinische Ophthalmologica* 216:261, 1981.

57. Milman, N., et al., "Lysine Prophylaxis in Recurrent Herpes Simplex Labialis," *Acta Dermatologica* (Stockholm) 60:85, 1980.

58. Myers, M., et al., "Failure of Neutral-Red Photodynamic Inactivation in Recurrent Herpes Simplex Virus Infections," *New England Journal of Medicine* 293:245, 1975.

59. Pasricha, J., "Ether Treatment of Herpes Simplex," *Archives of Dermatology* 107:775, 1973.

60. Pavan-Langston, D., et al., *Adenine Arabinoside: An Antiviral Agent.* New York: Raven Press, 1975 (425 pages).

61. Pazin, G., et al., "Prevention of Reactivated Herpes Simplex by Interferon," *New England Journal of Medicine* 301:325, 1979.

62. Rowe, N., et al., "Clinical Trial of Topical 3% Vidarabine Against Recurrent Herpes Labialis," *Oral Surgery* 47:142, 1979.

63. Skinner, G., et al., "Boric Acid Treatment for Cold Sores," *British Medical Journal,* September 22, 1979.

64. Spruance, S., "Ineffectiveness of Topical Ara-AMP in Recurrent Herpes Simplex Labialis," *New England Journal of Medicine* 300:1180, 1979.

65. Spruance, S., et al., "Treatment of Recurrent Herpes Simplex Labialis with Levamisole," *Antimicrobial Agents and Chemotherapy* 15:662, 1979.

66. Taylor, C., et al., "Topical Treatment of Herpes Labialis with Chloroform," *Archives of Dermatology* 113:1550, 1977.

67. Trousdale, M., et al., "Evaluation of Antiherpetic Activity of FIAC," *Investigative Ophthalmology* 21:826, 1981.

CYTOMEGALOVIRUS (CMV) AND THE GAY POPULATION

68. Bell, A., *Homosexualities: A Study of Diversity Among Men and Women.* New York: Simon & Schuster, 1978.

69. Cheeseman, S., et al., "Human Interferon-Effect on CMV and Herpes Simplex," *New England Journal of Medicine* 300:1345, 1979.

70. Durack, D., "Opportunistic Infections and Kaposi's Sarcoma in Homosexual Men," *New England Journal of Medicine* 305:1465, 1981.

71. Hyde, H. H., *The Love That Dares Not Speak Its Name.* Boston: Little, Brown & Co., 1970.

72. Ismach, J., "Health Hazards Among Homosexuals," *Medical World News,* p. 56, November 23, 1981.

73. Knox, G., "Comparative Prevalence of Subclinical Cytomegalovirus and Herpes Simplex Virus Infections in the Genital and Urinary Tracts of Low-Income Urban Women," *Journal of Infectious Disease* 140:419, 1979.

74. Lemon, S., et al., "Simultaneous Infection with Multiple Herpesviruses," *American Journal of Medicine* 66:270, 1979.

75. Sagihr, M., et al., *Male and Female Homosexuals: A Comprehensive Investigation.* Baltimore: Williams & Wilkins, 1973.

HERPES ZOSTER (shingles)

76. Brunnell, P., et al., "Zoster in Children," *American Journal of Diseases of Children* 115:432, 1968.

77. Chenitz, J., "Herpes Zoster in Hodgkin's Disease," *Journal of Dentistry in Children* 43:184, 1976.

78. Johnson, J., et al., "Herpes Zoster and Paralytic Ileus [painful stomach]," *British Journal of Surgery* 64:143, 1977.

79. Nally, F., et al., "Herpes Zoster of the Oral and Facial Structures," *Oral Surgery* 32:221, 1971.

GLOSSARY

ANTIBIOTIC A chemical substance either synthesized by man or produced by bacteria or fungi which has the capability to inhibit the growth of or to destroy bacteria or other germs.

ANTIBODY A type of serum protein (globulin) synthesized by white blood cells of the lymphoid type in response to an antigenic stimulus, the role of antibody being to inactivate or render harmless the invading antigen.

ANTIGEN A substance, usually protein or protein-sugar complex in nature, which, being foreign to the bloodstream or tissues of an animal, stimulates the formation of specific blood serum antibodies and white blood cell activity. Re-exposure to similar antigen will reactivate the white blood cells and antibody programmed against this specific antigen.

ANTIMETABOLITE A chemical structurally similar to one required for normal cellular functioning and metabolism; effect is exerted commonly by replacing or interfering with cellular use of the necessary normal metabolite.

ANTIVIRAL Any of a number of drugs or agents capable of destroying viruses or inhibiting their growth or multiplication until the body is capable of destroying the virus itself. Most antiviral drugs are members of the antimetabolite family.

BACTERIUM An infectious agent invisible to the naked eye but large enough to be seen with an ordinary laboratory microscope; capable of growing on nonliving nutrients; susceptible to members of the antibiotic family, such as penicillin and tetracycline.

BLISTER A localized collection of clear fluid causing elevation of the skin, separating it into an upper and lower layer. Breakdown of a blister produces an ulcer.

CARCINOMA IN SITU A tumor growth wherein the cells still lie within the very superficial surface cells of the skin or mucous membrane, without invasion to deeper tissues. Commonly descriptive of changes seen in the female uterine cervix in early malignant disease. Treatment is highly successful. (Abbreviated: CIS.)

CHROMOSOME The cellular DNA material which contains the genes or hereditary factors passed on from cell generation to cell generation.

CHICKEN POX An acute, highly infectious illness, principally of young children, caused by the chicken pox-herpes zoster virus and marked by fever and successive eruptions of clear blisters over the body. Chicken pox may enter latency in the deep nerve ganglia and reactivate years later in the form of herpes zoster.

CONVULSION A violent, involuntary series of contractions of the major muscles of one part or the entire body, due to abnormal stimulation of the brain by an irritating disease process.

CROSS-REACTIVITY A phenomenon seen in testing for specific blood antibodies against such organisms as herpes simplex type-1 and -2. The separate viruses have stimulated production of common or similar antibodies which cannot be distinguished from each other by reaction against the individual virus types.

CYTOMEGALOVIRUS A member of the herpes virus family which may induce the immune-deficient state or cause active illness, such as pneumonia, in a patient already immune-deficient due to chronic illness, such as cancer or organ transplantation therapy. (Abbreviated: CMV.)

CYTOPLASM The contents of a cell, exclusive of the nucleus.

DELUSION A logically founded but false belief which cannot be corrected by reasoning or persuading a person of the truth without the intervention of formal psychotherapy. Not always totally amenable to treatment but may be minimized.

DNA Deoxyribonucleic acid, the protein-sugar substance which contains the genetic information of any living cell.

ECZEMA A skin disease characterized by local patches of dryness and inflammation and often associated with immune-incompetence, such that patients are unable to mount a normal immune blood cell protection against invading infectious agents.

ENCEPHALITIS An infection or inflammation of the brain tissue itself, most commonly caused by viruses but may also be due to chemical irritation or nonspecific inflammatory or allergic illness.

EPIDEMIC An unusually sudden and high rise in the prevalence of any particular disease within the population.

ESOPHAGUS The mucous membrane tube connecting the back of the throat with the stomach.

EXTRAGENITAL Located outside of the genital region.

GANGLION A group of nerve cell bodies clustered together in a uniform mass outside of but often close to the brain or spinal cord. Nerves run to or from the ganglia in passage to or from the brain to specific sites on the body.

GONORRHEA A contagious, infectious venereal disease transmitted during sexual intercourse and caused by the bacterium *Neisseria gonorrhea*. Disease involves pain, odoriferous urine, and purulent discharge from the genitalia and widespread inflammation of the internal genital organs in both men and women.

HERPANGINA An infectious illness characterized by sudden onset of fever and blistering or ulceration in the mouth; caused by the coxsackie group of viruses, not related to herpes virus.

HERPES VIRUSES The viral family which includes the infectious agents of herpes simplex types 1 and 2, cytomegalovirus (CMV), and Epstein-Barr (mononucleosis) viruses. Herpes zoster is sometimes considered a member of this family because of the similar physical appearance, ability to infect the body chronically in latent state, and ability to cause one or more recurrent herpetic illnesses. It is usually characterized by blister and ulcer formation on the skin.

HERPES ZOSTER An acute, blistering, ulcerative, inflammatory illness of the skin caused by latent chicken pox virus migrating from the deep nerve ganglion to the zone of skin innervated by that nerve. Called also shingles, zoster, or zona.

IMMUNE-COMPETENT A person capable of mounting a full and normal white blood cell and antibody defense against invading foreign antigens such as viruses or bacteria.

IMMUNE-DEFICIENT A chronically ill patient who is incapable of mobilizing defensive white blood cells or antibodies against invading germs or other antigens.

INTERFERON A protein substance, formed by animal or other cells in interaction with viruses or certain chemicals, which is capable of conferring nonspecific resistance to infection with a wide range of viruses.

IRITIS Inflammation of the iris (blue or brown tissues near the front of the eye), with or without the presence of infection.

KERATITIS Inflammation of the cornea (clear window at the front of the eye), with or without associated infection.

LATENCY The state of apparent inactivity during which time the herpes virus genetic material lies sleeping in a cell without producing virus-specific biochemical changes or evidence of reproduction or illness; latent virus is not detectable by the usual biochemical tests.

MENINGITIS Infection or inflammation of the membrane surrounding the brain and spinal cord. Most commonly caused by bacteria but also by viruses, fungi, chemicals, or diffuse inflammatory illness of any kind.

MONONUCLEOSIS An acute, infectious disease caused by the herpes virus, Epstein-Barr virus, with fever and inflamed swelling of the lymph nodes around the neck, under the arms, and in the groin.

NONPRIMARY INFECTION A first infection in a particular location of the body, such as the genitalia, in a person who has had a previous infection with herpes virus elsewhere in the body and therefore has antiherpes antibody and white blood cells. This provides partial protection against the new herpes virus. (See also PRIMARY HERPES.)

NONVENEREAL DISEASE Any illness not due to or resulting from sexual activity. Most herpes infections are *not* venereal.

NUCLEUS A round body within a living cell and containing a number of functional subunits, among which are the chromosomes containing the genetic or hereditary information of the cell. Site from which many of the cell functions are directed.

ORAL-GENITAL Pertaining to contact between the mouth and genitalia during sexual activity.

PAP SMEAR Papanicolaou test: a smear of various body secretions, such as from the vagina or digestive tract, which is stained by the Pap stain in examination of the cells to detect various stages of the malignant process.

PHOBIA A persistent and abnormal dread or fear of an object or situation which normally would not stimulate such marked reactivation.

PLACENTA The blood-vessel-filled organ within the pregnant womb. It establishes communication between mother and baby by means of the umbilical cord for purposes of nutrition and the carrying away of wastes from the infant.

PRIMARY HERPES A first infection with either herpes simplex type-1 or type-2 virus in a person who has never previously been infected with either form of simplex. Antiherpes, antibodies, and white cells are absent and overt disease may or may not develop.

PROCTITIS Inflammation or infection of the rectal, anal, and perianal tissues; may be of venereal or nonvenereal origin.

REACTIVATION The change from a dormant or latent state to one of active growth and replication; with reference to herpes virus, the passage from latency to active infectious organisms resulting in recurrent illness.

RECOMBINANT DNA TECHNOLOGY The science of using the transfer of genetic material (DNA) to bacteria for the purpose of having those bacteria produce the chemical substance normally stimulated by the information programmed in the transferred DNA: e.g., insulin, interferon.

RECURRENT HERPES Repeated episodes of herpetic infectious blistering of the skin and mucous membrane due to reactivation of latent virus sleeping in the deep nerve ganglia which innervates that particular area of the body. Antiherpes antibodies and white cells are present but cannot totally prevent recurrent illness.

REINFECTION Reintroduction of an infectious agent from an outside source, as opposed to reactivation of an organism already residing in the body.

SARCOMA A tumor composed of closely packed cells which are highly immature in nature and malignant.

SYPHILIS A contagious venereal disease caused by a germ in the spirochete bacterial family and transmitted most commonly by direct sexual contact; causes a variety of deep tissue and skin sores which may come and go without therapy but which without treatment lead to severe body changes, including mental deterioration and blindness.

TZANCK SMEAR Similar in technique and purpose to a Pap smear.

ULCER A loss of the superficial layer of the skin or mucous membranes in a localized area, usually associated with redness, serous moisture, and irritation until scabbing occurs.

VAGINA The tubelike structure which extends from the external female genitalia to the cervix of the uterus (womb) and which serves as the birth canal during delivery and receives the penis during sexual intercourse.

VAGINITIS Inflammation or infection of the vagina.

VENEREAL DISEASE An illness or infection due to or enhanced by sexual activity.

VIRUS A minute infectious agent too small to be seen under the ordinary laboratory light microscope but visible under the magnification of the electron microscope. The individual particle consists of a central genetic (heredity) core made of DNA or RNA but not both. This is surrounded by a protein coat which may be multilayered. Some viruses, such as herpes, have a third coating which is membranous in nature and may be taken from the animal cell just infected. Viruses may infect animals, plants, or bacteria. They are not susceptible to the usual antibiotics, such as penicillin, but may be inhibited by special antimetabolites or other antiviral agents which have little to no effect on bacteria. Viruses are incapable of growing anywhere but within living cells.

VULVA The external (outside) female genital organ, including the major lips, minor lips, pubic mound, clitoris, perineum (region between vagina and rectum), and entry to the vagina.

WHITE BLOOD CELLS Those blood corpuscles responsible for maintaining the body's immune surveillance system against invasion by foreign substances such as viruses or bacteria. White cells become specifically programmed against foreign invaders and work to inactivate and rid the body of the foreign substance.

INDEX